Productivity for Live Entertainment and Theatre Technicians

Productivity Through Wellness for Live Entertainment and Theatre Technicians provides the tools for individuals and organizations to achieve a healthy work–life balance and increase productivity in the production process of live entertainment.

Through examination of the limits of the human body, the fundamentals of motivation, and best practices of project management, the reader will develop operational mindfulness and look at new ways to achieve work–life balance. The book explores case studies that show how organizations are promoting work–life balance and reaping the benefits of increased productivity, makes recommendations to reduce burnout and increase productivity among technicians, and discusses how to deal with the various phases of production.

An excellent resource for live entertainment technicians, production managers, technical directors, arts managers, managers in live entertainment, and students in Technical Direction and Production Management courses, *Productivity Through Wellness for Live Entertainment and Theatre Technicians* offers practical solutions to improve the quality of life of employees, reduce the burnout and injuries of overwork, and maximize the value of an hour.

Brian MacInnis Smallwood has been researching the impact of wellness on productivity since 2010. He has led workshops and seminars for Washington College, the Southeastern Theatre Conference, and the United States Institute for Theatre Technology. A cofounder of The Arts Wellness Group, Brian currently serves as an associate professor and production manager for the School of Theatre and Dance at James Madison University.

Productivity Through Wellness for Live Entertainment and Theatre Technicians

Increasing Productivity, Avoiding Burnout, and Maximizing the Value of an Hour

Brian MacInnis Smallwood

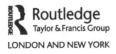
Routledge
Taylor & Francis Group

LONDON AND NEW YORK

First published 2020
by Routledge
52 Vanderbilt Avenue, New York, NY 10017

and by Routledge
2 Park Square, Milton Park, Abingdon, Oxon, OX14 4RN

Routledge is an imprint of the Taylor & Francis Group, an informa business

Library of Congress Cataloging-in-Publication Data
A catalog record for this title has been requested

ISBN: 978-0-367-13768-7 (hbk)
ISBN: 978-0-367-13770-0 (pbk)
ISBN: 978-1-003-00087-7 (ebk)

Typeset in Stempel Garamond LT Std
by Wearset Ltd, Boldon, Tyne and Wear

For my extended professional family. Yes, you.

Contents

Preface

When I started in this industry, I thought being a workaholic was a strength. My first production company was called "No Time for Love Productions," and it was aptly named. As I worked, I starved relationships, set aside dreams, and damaged my body. The thing is, I thought that was the only way to succeed.

I've since learned that I was not alone in that thinking. Many of us believe that the price to pay for working in theatre is to be a starving artist. To this day I discuss whether or not one can work in theatre and attend weddings, or have a spouse, or start a family. It seems the "starving artist" must be starved not only of food, but also of time and of love.

My time at the Yale School of Drama was pivotal in my change of thinking. During that time, the program trained us to examine and reexamine our decision-making and production processes. It was time for me to examine and reexamine my life, and there were high stakes in doing so. During those three years, I raised a baby boy and grew my family with a baby girl. I had to learn how to leave work at work to sustain the family.

My journey toward this topic began with a study of sleep deprivation. I could very much relate to the topic, as I was experiencing it at the time. As I explored and began to understand the boundaries of healthy sleep and how to improve my sleep habits, I adjusted my lifestyle and improved my quality of life. More importantly, I began to work more efficiently. I owe a lot to Bill Reynolds, my professor at the time and a dear colleague to this day, for pointing me in this direction.

When the time came to pick a thesis topic, I focused on the relationship between productivity and employee wellness. Much of what is in this book started with that thesis. I especially want to thank Bohdan Bushell and Randy Steffen for sharing their stories and contributing to the thesis. Two of my thesis interviewees asked to remain anonymous, and so I want to thank them as well (you know who you are, and how grateful I am for your contributions).

I also want to thank my readers, Jeff Wild (may he rest in peace) and Richard Girtain, for their positive feedback and encouraging review. I also wish to thank my reader Ash Bishop for reminding me not to get too presumptuous in my work. I also wish to honor the faculty at the Yale School of Drama who worked so patiently to ensure my matriculation, especially Ben Sammler, Alan Hendrickson, Jon Reed, Neil Mulligan, Don Harvey, Erich Bolton, and Elisa Cardone.

I also need to thank Mike Backhaus, Justin Bennett, Alex Bergeron, Joey Brennan, Nicole Bromley, Eric

Casanova, Ted Griffith, Ryan Hales, Nora Hyland, Kate Newman, Laura Patterson, Jon Pellow, Dan Perez, Hannah Shafran, Barbara Tan-Tiongco, Karen Walcott, and Jackie Young for their comradery when it was needed the most – gotta love those Technical Design & Production alums.

The notion of writing a book on this topic was made real by Stacey Walker and Lucia Accorsi at Routledge. The truth is that this book would not be here without their guidance and wisdom. Edward Weingart was an exceptional technical editor, and I greatly appreciate his feedback. I also want to thank Chelsea Pace, who served as a mentor in the application process. I especially want to thank Nils Emerson and Becky Merold for sharing their stories and contributing to the book.

I also want to thank all my dear friends for bouncing ideas around, challenging my logic, and supporting me through the process. Julia Surette, Laura "Nemesis" Eckelman, Robert Mahon, Dante Smith, Michael Stone, Ryan Kirk, Mel Johnston, and Jim Van Bergen among many others: thank you.

Perhaps most importantly, I want to thank my wife Rachel Smallwood, not only for her help with the illustrations and the cover but also for her patience, perspective, and love; and lastly, my children, Daniel Gordon Smallwood and Amelia Danger Smallwood, for reminding me that there is more to life than just work.

To you, the reader, I wish a happy and healthy life, and that you live to enjoy your retirement.

Introduction

Every manager, artist, and producer wants the same thing out of a production team: for everyone to do their best work. I translate this to mean that we want everyone involved to be as productive as possible.

As many books focus on the skills and tools necessary to enhance productivity, this book will focus on wellness and management techniques.

Writing a book on productivity and management in live entertainment undoubtedly raises some questions. "Who the hell are you to tell me what to do?" is one of those questions, as is "Why should I change what I'm doing?"

Combine that with the topic of personal and emotional burnout, and you get questions like "So, can you solve the burnout problem at my work?" and "Can you ease suffering right now?"

I would love to rattle off some amazing answers to these questions that quickly and succinctly inspire the reader and give utmost confidence that some shiny new technique will solve everything. Unfortunately, that would be the same as me saying "I have found the *one* true way to produce theatre, follow these steps." Such a statement would be ludicrous: there are too many variables, too many styles, too many players, and quite frankly, too many different desired outcomes to prescribe a single technique for production.

So, if the goal of this book is not to tell you what to do and how to do it, then what are we doing here?

Over my 20 years of production experience, I've noticed that many organizations are so caught up in what they are doing (building the set, altering the design, hitting deadlines) that they lose sight of how they are doing it. Each event becomes its own chapter in an organization's history. Whether the event is seen as good or bad, it seems completely isolated from the others. We start hearing statements like "You think this is bad, you should have been here for [enter show name here]." Perhaps it's even more generalized: "Well, we're not good at doing musicals, so get ready to stay late." Sometimes the "bad" is attributed to an individual or department, and everyone moves forward begrudgingly: "Oh, scenery is never on time, so get ready for some long nights."

Even if these statements are true, once these insights are voiced, the inquiry stops. It is logical in a way: why explore how the process is flawed if we know the result? The end starts to look like the means. It can also be really difficult to assess a previous production while in the midst of an aggressive schedule.

Without inquiry, however, there is no room for improvement. Bill Reynolds, my mentor in safety training, has often said: "Safety is a journey, not a destination." I think this statement can easily be adapted to organizational and individual productivity, as well as avoiding burnout. We need to constantly drill deeper into the question. I highly recommend my son's technique: just keep asking why.

"Well, we're not good at doing musicals."

Why?

"Because everyone works ridiculous hours."

Why?

And so on. Drill down and get to the base of the event and go from there.

I often say that everything has a strength and a weakness, and when it comes to analyzing your own organization, there is both a great advantage and a great disadvantage. The advantage is that no one knows your area better than you do. You know the variables, you know the processes, you have the institutional knowledge, and you have the most current understanding of what is going on.

The disadvantage is that it is often difficult to look at an organization critically when you are in it. This is why many companies do not know what their own competitive advantage is. Call it "not seeing the forest for the trees," but it can be very difficult to think pragmatically about a process that you are actively engaged in. Just try improving load in efficiency while also guiding a crew through the in-air installation of a 14,000-pound Jumbotron. It is going to be difficult to split focus.

We now get to the point of this book. The intention is to facilitate discussion and inquiry, and to share ideas regarding how to maximize the efficiency of an organization.

I should be clear that you need not be affiliated with a limited liability company, nonprofit, or corporation to be an organization. Perhaps the reader is a freelancer. Well, then, you are your own business, and an organization of one. Use this information to better manage your own time and resources to maximize your output and product quality, which will hopefully lead to more work, a higher quality of life, and a better work–life balance.

The book will address several different components of the production process that are often instinctively executed rather than practically assessed.

The "Working" section of the book outlines the forest. Less about the nuts and bolts of moving a project forward, this section talks about the modern workplace and how burnout and exhaustion can manifest. This section should also help provide data points you could use when starting the conversation within your own organization.

The "Motivation" chapter unpacks various factors that affect the productivity of workers, as well as different techniques and approaches for motivating your workforce. This section speaks to workplace satisfaction and can aid in retention and morale.

We will also discuss "The Human Body." Think of this as the manual for the tool that is the human body. We want to understand how to use it correctly without voiding the warranty, right? Similarly, this chapter will help the reader understand what limitations should be considered and how to safely push the envelope without doing harm.

"Managing the Work" provides tools and strategies to plan for the scope and scale of the work to be done. With practice and planning, one should be able to get ahead of most problems before they hit, thus mitigating burnout conditions.

And for those like my former classmate Alex Bergeron, who famously asked "Are we going to learn anything practical in this class?", the "Case Studies" chapter contains several personal perspectives that establish how different companies are applying these principles to meet the production needs of their clients.

For a large part of my career, I felt controlled by, or at least subject to, the production process. I felt carried along as if by the seas, and whether a process was smooth sailing or tumultuous and stormy, I had no agency in it. I was simply there to stand fast and do my job. My hope is that this book allows you, the reader, to question your own practices and make adjustments to improve your quality of life while doing your best work.

Chapter 1
Is This Even a Problem?

Working in the modern economy can seem relentless at times. Limited resources, tight deadlines, and low base wages all contribute to a need to work long hours. Indeed, many in live entertainment find the notion of working a 40-hour week laughably naïve. The issue of long work hours is not, however exclusive to one industry. Fire departments, trucking companies, hospitals, and the military are also wrestling with the question of productivity versus exhaustion.

The matter is deadly serious in these industries. Firefighters, for example, are more likely to die from cancer, cardiac arrest, or suicide due to exhaustion than in a fire.[1] These industries are the sources of extensive research, which is the foundation that this book draws from. That said, how widespread is the problem?

Japan

At the time of this writing, Japan has been in the news a lot lately due to exhaustion in the workplace. Partially due to a history of loyalty to company, but also due to a devalued entry-level workforce, the Japanese work scene is extremely taxing on its workers.[2] The situation has become so bad that business workers are regularly falling asleep in the street. Commonly, people will chalk outline the body to make it look like a crime scene.

Karōshi

That Japanese coined the term *Karōshi* in the early 1970s. Translated, it means "death by overwork."[3] This term is not used as hyperbole. It refers specifically to a literal death attributed to overwork. To help explain this issue further, consider two victims discussed by Chris Weller in the *Business Insider* article entitled "Japan is facing a 'death by overwork' problem – here's what it's all about."

Miwa Sado was a journalist working for the NHK news network in the summer of 2013. She reportedly worked 159 hours of overtime over the course of a month. Shortly afterward she died of heart failure. Ms. Sado was 31 years old.

Another form of *karōshi* is exemplified by Matsuri Takahasi. Ms. Takahashi worked 105 hours of overtime at the Dentsu advertising agency. On Christmas Day, she emailed her mother: "Work is unbearable. Life is unbearable. Thank you for everything[4]" before jumping off her employer's roof. Ms. Takahashi was 24 years old.

Let us consider the two instances of *karōshi* discussed above, but in smaller increments.

One hundred and fifty-nine hours of overtime, divided out over four weeks and added to a 40-hour work week, equals four 80-hour weeks. Assuming six days, that is a string of approximately 13.5-hour work days.

The 105 hours of overtime, calculated in the same way, equals four 66.25-hour weeks. Over six days, that is a string of 11-hour work days.

These seem like normal working hours to many of us.

These are not isolated incidents. The Japanese government reported 2,000 deaths due to overwork in one year back in 2016.[5] As of 2015, approximately 22 percent of the Japanese workforce clock more than 49 hours per week.[6] With a workforce population of 66.25 million (in 2015), that means about 14.58 million workers.

United States

On its surface, the US seems to be doing better at just 16 percent working over 49 hours per week,[7] but that percentage must be applied to a larger populace. In 2015, there were 321 million people in the country, and approximately 59.3 percent were in the workforce.[8] So, 59.3 percent of the population is about 190.35 million, 16 percent of which is 30.46 million people; that is more than double the number of people working overtime in Japan.

Live Entertainment

At the time of this writing, I have been unable to find a study that tracks how many hours live entertainment professionals work. I have found, anecdotally, that the hours tend to be well above 49 hours at different points in the process.

There are also grim implications that *karōshi* may be at work in our industry. The suicide rates in the live entertainment field, for example, are staggeringly high. In 2018, the Center for Disease Control found that the "Arts, design, entertainment, sports and media: jobs such as illustrators, designers, professional sports players and actors" occupational group had the second highest suicide rate among men, and *the* highest suicide rate among women.

While I do not mean to argue that all of those deaths can or should be attributed to exhaustion, I do believe that the matter is serious enough that more research is required.

Culture of Exhaustion

Given the industry demands for a constrained timeline, it is only natural that the workplace culture should adapt to support it. When the hours get long, technicians are told that "the show must go on." Over the course of my career in theatrical production, I have heard the expression countless times, usually in preparation for an aggressive load in or tech schedule. When I hear the statement, it is used as a rallying cry to encourage the production team to work through some complication or issue, often pushing the limits of exhaustion.

It turns out that using the expression to justify long work hours is inconsistent with the original intent. "The show must go on" was first used within the circus community in the nineteenth century. The expression meant that, should something go wrong in the performance, the ringmaster and band should keep the show going.[9]

Fundamentally, this expression is meant to be used during a performance, not in preparation for a performance.

To me, the frequent use of this expression over the years is an evolution of the workplace culture of live entertainment. Live entertainment seems to thrive on selfless acts that benefit the production. Perhaps a director dips into their own finances to help fund an otherwise unattainable prop. A technical director comes in after hours and works to bring a scenic element closer to completion. A costumer takes a project home to work on through the weekend. Some designers state that, for many companies, it is expected that they will use some of their "capital" to call in favors to keep the show in budget. These are all acts that are for the good of the show, but what about the impact on the worker?

It is my experience that nothing comes for free, even if there is no dollar sign attached, and these acts are no exception. These small acts of martyrdom start as honest gestures of commitment to a project, which is a beautiful thing. However, when this behavior is left unchecked and encouraged, the cost starts creeping in.

Robyn Melhuish's article "Work Martyrs Are Poisoning Your Culture"[10] discusses the impact of such a culture. She states that it can affect hiring/retention, productivity, and employee health. To help identify the presence of martyrdom in the workplace, she offers the following "Martyr Thoughts":

1. I can't take a day off of work.
2. Nobody can do my job except me.

3. I need to be constantly available for work.
4. I don't want to seem replaceable.

If you find those thoughts to be deeply relatable, you're not alone. Furthermore, I have worked at some organizations where this workplace culture has evolved into a business model.

This is problematic, as it can generate disgruntled employees. A report completed by the US Travel Association titled *The Work Martyr's Cautionary Tale* found that 47 percent of employees who are dissatisfied with their jobs believe that martyrdom in the workplace is a "good thing."[11]

The Manager's Agency

If your workplace embraces martyrdom, your employees are tacitly encouraged to overwork. There is risk associated with overwork, so the question becomes "What am I supposed to do about it?" This is usually where the conversation gets cyclical.

The manager says: "I can't control burnout in my employees, because I can't make them take care of themselves." What follows is a series of suggestions that the employee should focus more on self-care; eat right, get sleep, exercise, meditate, do yoga, or simply say "no" when the situation is too taxing. From the manager perspective, the employee has all the control.

When you talk to the employees, they say: "We can't possibly control burnout because the manager is asking too much of us." Then there are accusations that the company is taking on too much work for it to reasonably accomplish. Some lament that the hourly is too low, so they are taking extra work to make ends meet. Employees claim they have insufficient time and money to invest in self-care. There's usually a concern that saying "no" will be punished tacitly through reduced shifts or less desirable assignments. To the employee, the employer holds all the cards.

So, who's right? In my opinion, they're both right. This opinion is informed by the standards of The Occupational Safety and Health Administration (OSHA). Allow me to explain.

OSHA believes that there are two major parties responsible for creating a safe workplace: the employer and the employee. Briefly, the employer needs to establish safe work practices, reduce risk to the employee, maintain documentation, and train the employee. The employee needs to abide by safe practices, follow the training, and speak up regarding potential risks.

If the employer does their part, but the employee ignores training and doesn't wear the safety equipment, the likelihood of an accident goes up. Similarly, if the employee does what they are told, but the employer assigns dangerous tasks with no protections in place, someone is going to get hurt. It takes both parties committing to the same goal for this to work.

I believe the same principle can be applied to burnout and work–life balance. It is the employer's responsibility to manage the scope of the project so as to reduce the risk to the employee. This means scheduling with employee health in mind as well as allocating resources to ensure that everyone can do their best work. Furthermore, the employer should train employees about the risks of burnout as well as the resources/best practices to maintain work–life balance. The employee then needs to consider their schedules, maintain healthy habits, and use the resources available to maintain the balance.

Modelling

A manager carries a great deal of influence simply in what policy is enforced and how it is enforced. If a manager pays lip service to company priorities, but their actions demonstrate a different set of priorities, the manager may be implementing what is commonly called shadow policy.

It is important to understand the difference between policy and shadow policy. Policy is the very public, extremely overt method of operation. For example, a written employee handbook outlining the drug policy for a commercial scene shop would be policy. If everyone follows the procedures for work completion, then it's working. If there are a bunch of workarounds that circumvent the policy, those workarounds are considered shadow policy.

I see shadow policy manifest in little ways. Perhaps there is a policy that a rigger must be present to operate a lineset, and there is a need to fly a batten out to get scenery under it. The team decides that they don't want to lose the time to find the rigger, so they operate without the rigger. The shadow policy starts to form, and the new precedent is that simple lineset shifts can happen if time is short.

Regardless of your feelings on whether the action of the shadow policy in this example is appropriate, it illustrates that action speaks louder than words. If there is a rule, and it is not adhered to, the rule loses its impact.

In the case of work–life balance policy, actions definitely speak louder than words. If the manager says: "Just tell me upfront if you can't take a call," that's all well and good. If the manager has a reputation for never calling employees who turn down a call, then the shadow policy is "Take the call if you want to work."

Works Cited

"Dentsu's 'Power Harassment Hell'." *Japan Today*, 24 October 2016.

"Death by Overwork: Karoshi in Japan." *YouTube* , uploaded by Now This, 6 November 2017, https://youtu.be/Qp_KiDqfjGo. Accessed 1 April 2019.

McCurry, J. "Clocking Off: Japan Calls Time on Long-Hours Work Culture." *The Guardian*, 22 February 2015.

McCurry, J. "Japanese woman 'dies from overwork' after logging 159 hours of overtime in a month." *The Guardian*, 5 October 2017.

Melhuish, R. "Work Martyrs are Poisoning Your Culture." *Talent Management & HR*, 28 Nov. 2016, www.tlnt.com/ work-martyrs-are-poisoning-your-culture/. Accessed 8 April 2019.

Morgenstern, M. "Japan's Habits of Overwork Are Hard to Change." *The Economist*, 2 Aug. 2018, www.economist.com/

asia/2018/08/02/japans-habits-of-overwork-are-hard-to-change. Accessed 1 April 2019.

Rogers, James T. *The Dictionary of Cliches.* New York: Facts on File Publications, 1985.

"The Work Martyr's Cautionary Tale." *U.S. Travel Association*, www.ustravel.org/research/work-martyr%E2%80%99s-cautionary-tale-how-millennial-experience-will-define-america%E2%80%99s-vacation. Accessed 8 April 2019.

Toomey, J. T. "Addicted to Awake: Sleep Deprivation in the Fire Service." Fire Engineering, 15 November 2018, www.fireengineering.com/2018/11/15/196617/addicted-to-awake/#gref. Accessed 1 April 2019.

United States Department of Labor, Bureau of Labor Statistics. (2016, June 7). "Employment–population ratio, 59.7 percent; unemployment rate, 4.7 percent in May." *TED: The Economics Daily*, 7 June 2016, www.bls.gov/opub/ted/2016/employment-population-ratio-59-point-7-percent-unemployment-rate-4-point-7-percent-in-may.htm?view_full. Accessed 1 April 2019.

Notes

1 (Toomey)
2 (Morgenstern)
3 ("Death by Overwork")
4 ("Dentsu's 'Power Harassment Hell'")
5 (McCurry, "Japanese Woman 'Dies from Overwork'")
6 (McCurry, "Clocking Off")
7 (McCurry, "Clocking Off")
8 (United States Department of Labor, Bureau of Labor Statistics)
9 (Rogers)
10 (Melhuish)
11 ("The Work Martyr's Cautionary Tale")

Chapter 2
Motivation

I worked with a colleague who would toil doggedly for a good independently produced Off-Off Broadway production. Whether it was long hours, poor working conditions, inclement weather, or illness, nothing would slow the steady drive to get a new work onto the stage. This was one of the hardest-working technicians I have ever worked with, and their productivity was unmatched.

When it came to the higher-paying Off-Broadway gigs, it was a different story. No-Call-No-Show[1] was common, attitude was dismissive, and work was accomplished begrudgingly. In time, I learned that this technician's productivity correlated with the perception that a project was "artful" or "important," and productivity was terrible if the project was deemed too "commercial."

To discuss wellness and productivity in the absence of motivation is like trying to assess ocean conditions without testing the water. In this section, we will explore what drives employees to increase productivity. Once we understand the rules of motivation, we can better determine how employee wellness affects motivation.

Motivation is heavily researched in the corporate world with a focus on employee retention and morale. For theatre and live entertainment, one can literally see the difference between a well-motivated and a poorly motivated workforce. Motivation during the load in and tech process likely impacts the number of notes achieved and thus the level of polish achieved for the performance.

The Potential of Productivity

One of the least quantifiable aspects of productivity is employee motivation. There are as many variables in the assessment as there are people to assess. That said, there are some similarities and guidelines that have come through polling and anthropological analysis to help managers improve productivity.

Factors

A study entitled "Speaking Out: What Motivates Employees to Be More Productive," initiated by Joshua Freedman and Carina Fiedeldey-Van Dijk, assessed what human factors affect productivity. Gender, race, age, and experience all had little to no impact. When asked whether or not an employee could be more productive, 97 percent reported in the affirmative. In fact, 20 percent reported they could double or triple productivity. With that kind of potential, what do employees need to get motivated?

The study highlighted seven primary factors for increasing productivity. In descending order of importance, they are:

- Reassurance
- Workplace climate

- Workplace skills
- Connectedness
- Intrapersonal factors
- Reward
- Resources

Reassurance

I once spoke with a director who said that the first/best step toward a good production process is learning literally everyone's name. The director understood the power of recognition.

Assurance, recognition, and positive reinforcement are the most sought-after factors by an employee.[2] These factors are connected to a sense that the work being done matters, and that the employee's contribution is valued. The study went on to say that warm feelings in employees are important for increasing productivity.

In live entertainment terms, one can understand how much better it feels to work for a grateful client rather than one that does not value your contribution. It is my experience that the production team will work harder for a designer who is appreciative than for one who treats the team as hired help or somehow "lesser" (see Figure 2.1).

Workplace Climate

Workplace climate could be translated to mean workplace culture. Dan Denison, PhD defines workplace culture as

> *The underlying values, beliefs and principles that serve as a foundation for an organization's management*

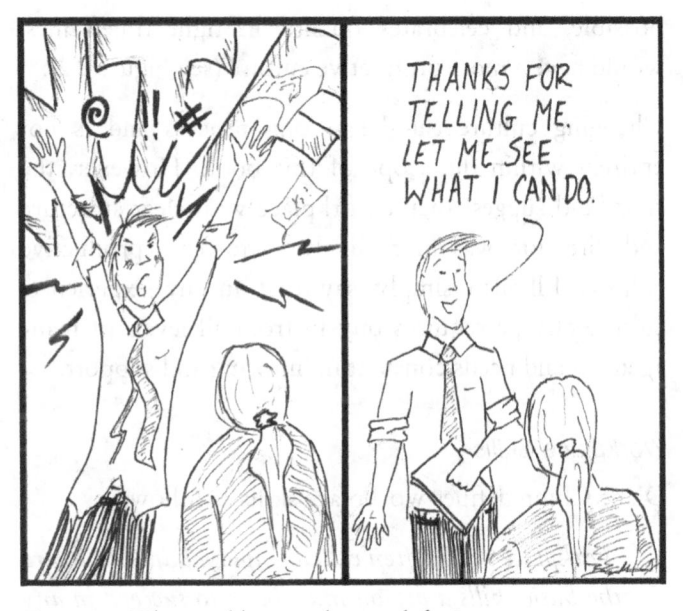

Figure 2.1 Who would you rather work for?

system as well as the practices and behaviors that both exemplify and reinforce those basic principles.[3]

A culture that is conducive to getting work done will, not surprisingly, inspire more productivity than a hostile one.

I see symptoms of workplace culture problems when discussing payment structures. I hear salaried workers saying: "We're paid the same anyway, so why try?" or hourly employees saying: "Don't work so fast, we're paid by the hour!" These are examples of a workplace culture that does not value productivity. A venue that encourages employees to work as quickly as is safely possible, and celebrates quality in tight timeframes, would have a more productive culture (see Figure 2.2).

Changing culture can be a long process and is not entirely within the scope of this book. However, the study did suggest that a workplace with clear structure and direction was more likely to foster a productive culture. I'll also simply say that in my experience, culture change requires buy-in from all levels of management and needs constant monitoring and support.

Workplace Skills

Diane Chinn defines workplace skills as follows:

> *Workplace skills, often called employability skills, are the basic skills a person must have to succeed in any workplace. They are the core knowledge, skills and attitudes that allow workers to understand instructions, solve problems and get along with co-workers and customers.*[4]

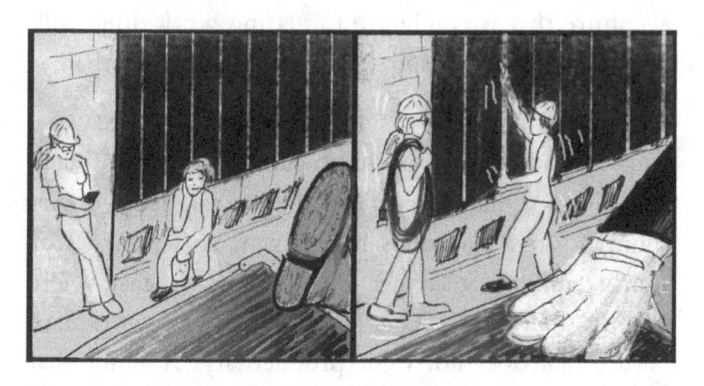

Figure 2.2 Where would you rather work?

To be clear, developing workplace skills enhances the productivity of the employees, not the supervisor. While any supervisor would benefit from these skills, a technical manager should think in terms of developing these abilities within an employee workforce to maximize efficiency.

Joshua Freedman and Carina Fiedeldey-Van Dijk found that the highest-rated skills were time management and focus. This makes sense, doesn't it? Time management means that less time is lost due to unclear priorities or incomplete planning. Enhanced ability to focus means less loss of efficiency due to distractions or reactions.

If there is less wasted time, and we are more focused during that time, it follows that the efficiency will lead to productivity. It should be noted that career development through continuing education was also seen as an important influence.

Connectedness

This refers to a sense of inclusion and cooperation with peers. When working on a team, being ostracized can wreak havoc on one's desire to work. If the employee is being shunned due to lack of productivity, this can become a self- sustaining cycle.

In addition, connectedness is a factor between supervisor and employee. If a manager does not trust or empower the employee, the need to micromanage and "do it myself" will greatly hinder the manager's ability to tackle their own tasks. If a worker feels they cannot go to the supervisor with questions or concerns, it creates an environment more prone to errors and wasted resources.

Intrapersonal Skills

Intrapersonal skills, as opposed to interpersonal skills, are about personal satisfaction. This is all about how the worker feels about their own work: feeling that the work is important, and that the employee sees self-value.

A desire for more responsibility, for example, represents a desire to take ownership as well as a confidence in one's own work. The ability to enjoy the work is another intrapersonal skill and is very important to motivation.

For example, I once met a scenic designer who was working on a production of *Oklahoma*! The director had no interest in the production – it was just a paycheck – and so they did not provide a concept or inspiration for the creative team. The designer worked hard to find elements of their own design to get excited about in an attempt to self-motivate.

Reward

Finally we get to money. Many may be surprised that more money, benefits, and other remunerative influences are the sixth most referenced factor. In 2011, Google polled its employees and found that financial compensation was not as important to its employees as a good relationship with their supervisor.[5]

Now, Google pays in the top 25 percent of its industry, so clearly the executives understand the value of paying employees. I think it is important to understand that the pay scale must feel "fair" to other similar positions in the market.[6] That said, many people entering the workforce value their own time more than money (see Figure 2.3).[7]

Resources

Productivity is affected by the equipment available. A high-precision scene shop that operates without a computer numerical control (CNC) router is likely to become more productive by acquiring one. Yes, there would be training involved, and yes, the initial use would probably not be as efficient, but in the long term, there is likely to be increased productivity.

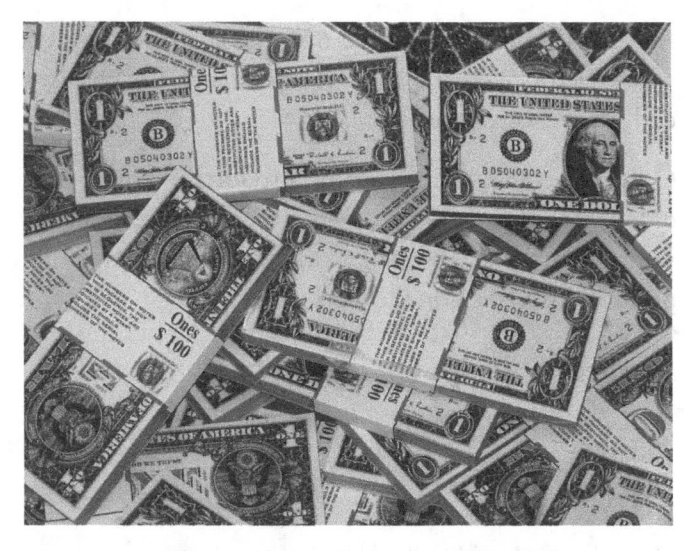

Figure 2.3 I wish I could give all of you a million dollars and free up more of your time. For now, this is the best I can do.

Having the tools, materials, and financial means to do the job quickly and effectively has an impact on potential productivity.

Different Workers and Different Factors

Freedman and Fiedeldey-Van Dijk's study revealed that 97 percent of employees studied reported that they could be more productive at work. However, the employees were performing at various levels of productivity and thus were influenced by different factors.

Low-level producers are more influenced by reassurance and reward. These are commonly entry-level employees who are just figuring things out, but they could also be disillusioned workers. Positive feedback and team inclusiveness are the kinds of reassurance cited.

Mid-level producers were all over the chart in terms of which factors were in play, but reassurance was consistently at the top of the list.

Only the most exceptionally productive employees didn't feel the need for reassurance. Top producers wanted efficiency through workplace skills and more personal investment in the work.

Productivity Tactics

> *I uh, I don't like my job, and uh, I don't think I'm going to go anymore.*
>
> *Peter from "Office Space"*

Now that we've identified the factors that can improve productivity, the question remains: how do we influence these factors in our employees? There have been a great many articles addressing management style, will, drive, and company policy. Looking at those articles through the lens of productivity potential, one can start to understand how the factors play into different management tactics.

Feedback

The Hawthorne Effect, first measured in Chicago at the Hawthorne Power Plant in 1924, is a phenomenon suggesting that workers are more productive when under observation.[8] When extrapolated, this suggests that an employee will be more productive if the worker perceives that the supervisor is invested in the employee's productivity. Some methods of feedback include the following.

Evaluation Meetings

Evaluations are an opportunity to set goals for an employee and provide feedback. This opportunity for feedback is why Google has gone so far as to institute weekly one-on-one meetings between supervisors and all staff members.[9] The benefit is that, over time, employees become more comfortable interacting with a supervisor and are more likely to speak freely rather than trying to answer in a way that pleases the supervisor.

Many theatres use "post-mortem" meetings to evaluate project success and create opportunities to improve. This is similar to the military's use of a mission debriefing or After Action Review (AAR). It can be very effective from both an operations and an individual wellness perspective.

In the Moment

More actionable feedback should be given as quickly as possible. That might not be in the middle of load in, but at a break or at the end of the day would be feasible.

Simply saying "good job" or "work harder" isn't specific or actionable. Discuss what the employee did to contribute toward the success of a project. Ask for ideas on how it could have gone even better. When giving constructive criticism, focus on how expectations weren't met and discuss strategies to ensure success next time. Don't let the need for constructive conversation fester, as it could become the "elephant in the room" if left alone, as shown in Figure 2.4.

Consider Your Relationship

"Praise publicly and criticize privately" is a great place to start when it comes to reassurance. Praising publicly not only highlights the individual accomplishment but also communicates to the team what a success looks like to management. Be sure to diversify the praise recipient, lest you create a sense of favoritism.

When criticizing privately, it may not be wise to be alone. In this litigious age, it is often recommended to have another supervisor in the room or to meet in a public place away from other employees. This will reduce the chance of slander or impropriety after the meeting is over.

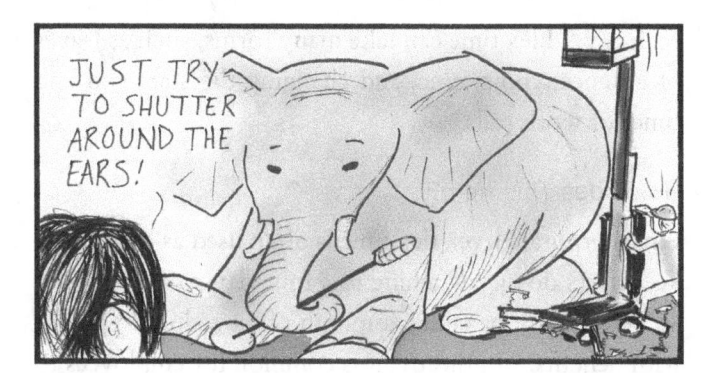

Figure 2.4 Ask any zookeeper: elephants affect productivity.

Feedback Versus Factors

In terms of our factors, what does this tactic give us? Regardless of whether it is praise or criticism, the evaluation shows that the employer is working toward keeping the employee effective. If handled correctly, this attention can be reassuring and contributes to a focused and goal-specific workplace environment. Connectedness will come over time, provided that all employees get a review (as opposed to singling out staff when something goes wrong). Achieving goals set by the employee and the supervisor will increase a sense of workplace satisfaction and may also be grounds for raises or promotions. If it is done properly, a supervisor can enhance five of seven factors to encourage productivity.

Flex Time

The Random House Dictionary defines flex time as "a system of working that allows the employee to choose, within limits, the hours for starting in and leaving work each day." Flex time can take many forms, such as leaves of absence, comp time, and changing the start and end times of work calls.

How Does This Help?

On a corporate level, flex time is often used as a means to keep costs down: switching to a four-day work week for 80 percent pay or taking a month off at reduced pay but with benefits.[10] In theatre, it is common for employees to work seasonal contracts rather than 12 months to reduce costs off season. This contract management is a way of implementing flex time.

Another option is to allow employees flexibility in scheduling. Giving employees control over their own schedules generally increases motivation and commitment. This translates into reduced instances of absenteeism.[11] In addition, it has been found that employees making use of flex time get more sleep and live healthier lifestyles.[12] In theatre, actors covet employment that is flexible enough to accommodate the need to leave for a production or audition.

So, Who's In Today?

One of the troublesome aspects of flex time is that it is sometimes difficult to coordinate. A supervisor may find the shop understaffed at a key time or that the person who served as a lead on a project is not there to relay a progress report. It's therefore important for a supervisor to establish protocols and objectives so that work does not grind to a halt.

That said, many companies ask the employees to establish the protocols that work per department. Allowing costume construction technicians to find the right solution for the costume shop will likely result in a more effective policy.

Flex Time Versus Factors

Giving an employee the ability to manage a work schedule is definitely an increase in responsibility. It's also a sign of trust. This would suggest that flex time promotes intrapersonal skills. In addition, the individual will need to develop his or her own systems of organization and time management to achieve goals while at the office. That counts toward workplace skill development.

Reassurance and connectedness would seem to suffer in this model. Reward may also take a hit with this tactic, as employees may not receive training or be seen as serious about the work.[13] This suggests that flex time would be a stronger motivator for high-productivity employees and that buy-in from the top would be essential.

Flexplace

"Flexplace refers to a company policy or program that enables employees to have more decision authority on where they will work regardless of time of day."[14] Often referred to as telecommuting, flexplace allows an employee to work off site; commonly from home.

How Does This Help?

The advantage of this kind of program is a potential increase in productivity. An employee with fewer distractions can stay more focused on the work. In addition, a suitable employee need not live within a commutable distance, so the hiring pool can be much broader. This arrangement can reduce overhead costs, as the employee is using fewer company resources to get the job done.[15]

Great, I'll Build the Show from Home

In theatre, this type of benefit can only work in very specific instances. It would be difficult to imagine an electrician hanging and focusing an instrument from home.[16] However, draftspersons, artisans with small projects, and customer service representatives could conceivably take advantage of flexplace.

The corporate world warns that the biggest challenges with this system involve isolation of an employee. Communication may fall off, leaving the employee feeling left behind. Employees also commonly overwork due to an inability to separate work life from home life.[17] Live entertainment professionals often omit information when communicating with other departments while working onsite. One could imagine how a flexplace employee could be more susceptible to this form of miscommunication.

Many live entertainment organizations use software such as Basecamp, Slack, and Propared to mitigate miscommunication.

Flexplace Versus Factors

The advantages and disadvantages of flexplace are akin to those of flex time, but amplified. The trust and responsibility required further enhance intrapersonal skills, and the regimented system for even basic communication grows workplace skills.

The employee may require more reassurance about being a valued team member. Scheduling quarterly meetings or setting days for the employee to report in to the workspace will help alleviate the sense of isolation.[18]

Job Sharing

This practice involves two workers splitting one full-time job, receiving salary and benefits commensurate with the amount of work done. This practice is common for those working through a medical leave or for those easing into retirement.[19]

I've Never Heard of a Theatre Trying This

This practice is only recently gaining momentum. It is far more common for an organization to hire a new employee to ease pressure on an overworked employee. That said, if an employee is buckling under the strain of a large workload, falls ill and can't do the same work as before, or has an opportunity to work another gig, this tactic could be applied.

Furthermore, it is very common for technical directors to hire in freelance draftspersons to help with the technical design elements of a production. If the payment is pulled from the technical director's fee, this is a form of job sharing.

Pitfalls

One common challenge with this practice is favoritism to full-time employees. Job sharers may face less training and opportunity for advancement. Supervisors must ensure steady communication between the two co-sharers and must keep a steady eye on the morale of the workplace.[20]

Job Sharing Versus Factors

This practice develops workplace skills and intrapersonal factors. The catch is that the employee whose job is split will take a pay cut. This is a tactic probably best used for specific circumstances that cater to an employee's need for a better work–life balance.

Natural Light

A recent study has found that melatonin and cortisol levels are higher in people exposed to natural rather than artificial light. This translates into higher levels of alertness and cognitive thinking. After six hours of exposure for two days, researcher Miirjam Münch found that the type of light "had an impact on cognitive task performance in the evening." She went on to suggest: "Such a relationship could be crucial for workers requiring high attention levels and executive functioning, such as bus drivers, industrial workers in sensitive areas, or air-traffic control."[21]

For live entertainment, many positions require high attention levels and executive functioning, including automation technicians, riggers, stage managers, and any other technicians who carry high-risk responsibilities when working nights. Finding ways to expose theatre employees to natural light when not working outdoors may take some creative thinking: perhaps using sunlight lamps in work lights for work calls.

If a supervisor has a say in the construction or renovation of a new building, it may be worth incorporating windows with blackout curtains, for example: anything that might bring more natural light into the workplace.

Natural Light Versus Factors

The only factor this seems to impact is workplace climate, but as that is the second most influential factor, this strategy is well worth considering. One might argue that oxygen only impacts workplace climate, but I sure wouldn't want to work somewhere without it.

Does This Touchy Feely Stuff Really Work?

In 1998, the Families and Work Institute initiated a study entitled "Business Work-Life Study," which surveyed over 100 companies. The survey found that employees who perceive that they are working in an organization that supports a work–life balance are more likely to feel invested in the company's success. These employees felt a strong sense of job satisfaction and were more loyal to the organization.[22]

There is evidence that many leaders of organizations see work-family programs as a zero-sum game in which "every time an employee's personal interests 'win,' the organization pays the price in its bottom line."[23] As managers, we can support these employees as individuals and adjust policy or strategy to suit each issue. The study generated some steps a manager can take to make quantifiable improvements.

Flexibility Instead of Reduced Workload

The researchers developed a 1–5 rating system for employees to gauge flexibility in the organization. The results showed that "implementing flexibility programs sufficient to improve employee perception of flexibility by 1 point on a 5-point flexibility scale is statistically equivalent to reducing workload by 11 hours per week per employee as related to perception of improving work-family balance."[24] This means no reduction in work hours with a better chance for increased productivity.

Adjust Manager Expectation

It is common to find managers who believe that "face-time" is a marker of productivity. It is important to change the mentality to focus on a "results-oriented" approach. Evaluation based on quantifiable goals rather than attendance can be a big culture adjustment, so plan accordingly and actively craft the rubric with which to measure a position.

Consider All Employees

The struggle to achieve work–life balance is extremely common with employees who have families. Historically, many managers have stereotyped women as the most in need of assistance in achieving balance. The study supports that the struggle is not limited on a gender basis and that "[t]he need for work-family balance and the benefits of flexibility are equally applicable to men and women." The study went on to conclude as follows:

> In summary, the results of this study indicate that perceived flexibility in the timing and location of work offers the promise of enabling employees opportunities to better balance work and family life in this era of increasing workload. These offerings appear to be true win-win solutions to help mitigate the personal toll of increased work demands. If visionary business leaders and empowered individuals adopt greater flexibility, we may see the end to the "zero-sum game" (Friedman et al., 1998) and set up a "virtuous cycle" in which work-family balance programs leverage on each other to promote individual well-being, family solidarity, and organizational success.

The Positive

At this point, it should make sense that a company that values its employees will foster motivation. Remember that fostering motivation is a lot like maintaining a long-running show; it takes constant inspection and maintenance.

I encourage you, good reader, to remember that the strength of a company is its people, and to remind the team that their contribution is valued.

Works Cited

Chinn, D. "The Definition of Workplace Skills." *Bizfluent*, 26 September 2017, https://bizfluent.com/info-7786830-definition-workplace-skills.html. Accessed 19 November 2019.

"Flexplace." *Wikipedia*, n.d. Accessed 28 March 2013.

Freedman, Joshua and Carina Fiedeldey-Van Dijk. "Speaking Out: What Motivates Employees to Be More Productive." CGI Conference, 2004, pp. 1–6.

Friedman, Stewart D. et al. "The Zero-Sum Game." *Harvard Business Review*, 1998, pp. 119–129.

GoodTherapy. "Does Natural Lighting Make Us More Productive?" *GoodTherapy blog*, goodtherapy.org/blog/natural-lighting-increases-productivity-0104112/, 4 January 2012. Accessed 2 April 2013.

Hanly, Samantha. "Description of Workplace Culture." *Chron*, n.d. https://smallbusiness.chron.com/description-workplace-culture-13379.html. Accessed 2 March 2020.

Hewlett, Sylvia Ann. "Making Flex Time a Win-Win," *The New York Times*, 12 December 2009, www.nytimes.com/2009/12/13/jobs/13pre.html. Accessed 27 March 2013.

Kovary, Giselle. "Job Sharing & Flex Places: Alternative Work Schedules for All Generations," *N-Gen blog*, 6 December 2012, www.ngenperformance.com/blog/hr-training/job-sharing-flex-places-alternative-work-schedules-all-generations. Accessed 27 March 2013.

"Light Work." *The Economist*, 4 June 2009, www.economist.com/finance-and-economics/2009/06/04/light-work. Accessed 27 March 2013.

Mr. 4HWD. "Why I Don't Work Over Time (Usually)." *The Four Hour Workday*, 25 February 2014. www.thefourhourworkday.com/why-i-dont-work-over-timeusually/. Accessed 18 November 2018.

Nayab, N. "Does a Flex Time Policy Result in Fewer Employee Absences," *Bright Hub*, 18 May 2011, www.brighthub.com/office/entrepreneurs/articles/75522.aspx. Accessed 27 March 2013.

Parker-Pope, Tara. "Does Flex Time Lead to Better Health?" *New York Times*, 12 December 2007. well.blogs.nytimes.com/2007/12/13/does-flex-time-lead-to-better-health/?mtrref=www.google.com&gwh=EC668005B594EA5924B1E0343591CA1C&gwt=pay&assetType=REGIWALL. Accessed 27 March 2013.

Rypple (Daniel Debow). "5 Ways to Keep Your Rockstar Employees Happy," *GigaOm*, 15 October 2011, https://gigaom.com/2011/10/15/5-ways-to-keep-your-rockstar-employees-happy/. Accessed 3 March 2020.

Wharton University of Pennsylvania. "Balancing the Pay Scale: 'Fair' vs. 'Unfair'," 22 May 2013, *Knowledge@Wharton*, knowledge.wharton.upenn.edu/article/balancing-the-pay-scale-fair-vs-unfair/. Accessed 18 November 2018.

Notes

1 The unfortunate practice of missing work when scheduled while also not communicating that the absence is coming.
2 (Freedman and Fiedeldey-Van Dijk)
3 (Hanly)
4 (Chinn)
5 (Rypple)
6 (Wharton University of Pennsylvania)
7 (Mr. 4HWD)
8 ("Light Work") The article goes on to question the effect, suggesting that the increase in productivity may be in large part due to exposure to natural lighting.
9 (Rypple)
10 (Hewlett)
11 (Nayab)
12 (Parker-Pope)
13 (Kovary)
14 ("Flexplace")
15 (Kovary)
16 Though, as technology improves ....
17 (Kovary)

18 (Kovary)
19 (Kovary)
20 (Kovary)
21 (GoodTherapy)
22 (Hewlett)
23 (Hewlett)
24 (Friedman et al.)

Chapter 3
The Human Body

A student once walked into my office and talked about leaving a job as an electrician at a local live event company. This young professional said the work had become more and more difficult and bemoaned how much easier the job had been a year prior. I asked about the work schedule; the student had spent the entire year working 60-hour weeks while also attending classes. He worked even longer hours when on school breaks.

Some say "Hey, I'm not a machine," but I disagree. We are machines, and just like any mechanical device, we require care to maximize our productivity. Our fuel supply must be replenished, our fluid levels must be maintained, and if we can say it with a straight face, we have a duty cycle. In the case of this student, the body had worked optimally at the beginning, but had run too hot for too long without recovery. The working hours exceeded the duty cycle.

This chapter consolidates information about two key factors that greatly impact burnout: stress and sleep. The more deeply we understand the needs of the system, the better we can maintain it.

Stress

The definition of stress that this book will address is: "mental, emotional, or physical strain or tension."[1] With such a broad definition, it should come as no surprise that every industry wrestles with stress. Medical, military, corporate, and legal occupations have studied the causes and impact of stress. What follows is extrapolated with an eye to live entertainment.

How Does Stress Work?

Robert Ostermann, professor at Fairleigh Dickinson University's Teaneck-Hackensack Campus, discusses how stress can be of great use. "No one reaches peak performance without being stressed, whether an athlete, an office worker, or a manager."[2] Rebecca Maxon sums up the idea in her article "Stress in the Workplace: A Costly Epidemic":

> *The natural pattern of human behavior is to experience a stress-causing event or situation, react to it with increased tension and return to a normal, relaxed state. The problem occurs when stress is so overwhelming or constant that this pattern is broken.*

(See Figure 3.1)

The Theories of Hans Selye

Hans Selye (1907–1982) is largely responsible for the influential theories that guide stress treatment at the time of this writing. It was Selye who first applied the term

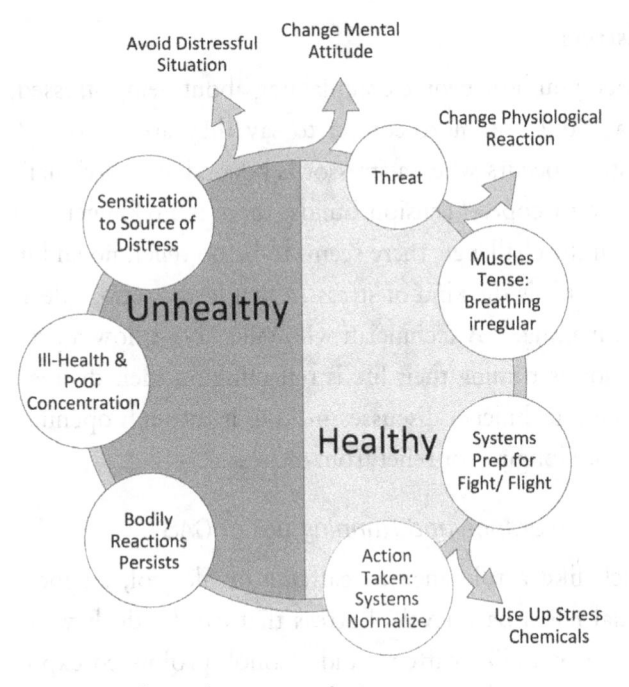

Figure 3.1 The cyclic process of stress.

"stressor" to describe human response to threat.[3] He also qualified stressors into Eustress and Distress.

Eustress

Eustress is positive stress that serves as a motivator.[4] Commonly referred to as "good stress," this is the stress that comes with facing conflict head on or achieving difficult goals. When theatre technicians talk about how rewarding cruise gigs are, they are reflecting on eustress. When technicians decide to leave a job because they do not feel challenged anymore, they are experiencing a lack of eustress.

Distress

When you hear people complaining about being stressed, they would be more correct to say they are distressed. Distress occurs when a stressor is beyond an individual's ability to cope. "Tension builds, there is no longer any fun in the challenge, there seems to be no relief, no end in sight. This is the kind of stress … that leads to poor decision making."[5] A technician who talks about how a production is ruining their life is reflecting on their distress. When a technician discusses making it through opening, they are longing for relief from distress.

Stress Tolerance and Running out of GAS

Much like a tolerance to caffeine or alcohol, an individual has a base level of stress that can be dealt with. However, unlike caffeine and alcohol, prolonged exposure to stressors erodes stress endurance rather than strengthening it.[6] Think of stress as a sensitizer or an allergy. The more often you are exposed, the weaker your resistance becomes.

Hans Selye studied the hormonal patterns associated with coping with stress. The "General Adaptive Syndrome" or "GAS" contains three stages. "Alarm" is the "fight or flight" stage where the body engages a threat. Dr. Lisa of the *Doctor-Recommended-Stress-Relief* blog clarifies:

> *At the level of eustress, we are faced with a challenge, we make a choice and we live with the consequences. Period. End of Story.*

The alarm stage lasts for seconds, but equalizing afterward may take minutes.[7] Consider hearing the bang from a heavy load drastically shifting in a poor truck pack. The loud noise it makes is startling, but the brain quickly assesses that there is no danger, and it then takes some time to calm down.

If, however, the stressful situation does not resolve quickly, that is, within seconds, Selye tells us that the body moves to the "resistance" stage. Again, Dr. Lisa:

> *The longer we have to cope with a situation, the more resources it demands on our body. Eventually we feel the effects of fatigue.*

To make this relatable, imagine a technician is working and someone gets hurt. The initial jolt or alarm phase takes moments; then the body adapts to the situation and the employee can apply training protocols and try to deal with the situation. After tending to the injury, filling out the paperwork, and getting to and from the hospital, the technician will likely feel that it has been a long and tiring day.

Finally, should the stress continue unmitigated, the body goes into "exhaustion," more commonly known as "chronic stress" or "burnout."[8] At this point, one's adaptation energy is depleted, and the individual cannot effectively deal with the stress any longer. The only healthy option at this point is to remove either the individual or the stressor from the situation.[9]

Durations of Stress

Hans Selye theorized that the amount of adaptation energy we have is finite, and we can only deal with so much stress.[10] If Selye is correct, then the duration of stress is extremely important. The following categories are established in a book entitled *The Stress Solution* by Lyle H. Miller, PhD, and Alma Dell Smith, PhD.

Acute Stress

This is the most common duration, and it stems from recent events. One goes from a sort of exhilaration to lethargy. For example, consider a first-time arena rigger tackling a note 100 feet above the deck. At first, the height and challenge cause adrenaline and endorphins to dump in the system, and the technician experiences some exhilaration and alertness. However, upon coming back down, the rigger may feel sluggish and want a break.

> *Because it is short term, acute stress does not have enough time to do the extensive damage associated with long-term stress ... Acute stress can crop up in anyone's life, and it is highly treatable and manageable.*[11]

Episodic Acute Stress

This category reflects unchecked acute stress. This is often seen in those with poor work–life balance. Workaholics, the unassertive, and anatidaephobics[12] often face episodic acute stress. Again, doctors Miller and Smith:

> *The symptoms of episodic acute stress are the symptoms of extended over arousal: persistent tension*

headaches, migraines, hypertension, chest pain, and heart disease. Treating episodic acute stress requires intervention on a number of levels, generally requiring professional help, which may take many months.

These are the technicians who are so used to being strung out, upset, and depressed that it becomes who they are. They often deny their own agency in situations, blaming creatives or area heads for their woes. To these worn-down individuals, the world is a stressful place. This is a very difficult position to get out of, as the technician does not see an exit in sight.

One can imagine how difficult it would be for a manager to change a culture where acute stress is pervasive. Doctors Miller and Smith suggest that the only lever to lean on to enact change is the promise of relief; however, their context is therapy. It is extremely dangerous for an untrained manager to attempt to play therapist in this environment. It is far better to refer the employee to a mental health professional.

Chronic Stress

To ensure that the reader does not underestimate the importance of chronic stress, the following excerpts are directly quoted from the American Psychological Association's website:

While acute stress can be thrilling and exciting, chronic stress is not. This is the grinding stress that wears people away day after day, year after year. Chronic stress destroys bodies, minds and lives. It wreaks havoc through long-term attrition. It's the stress of poverty, of dysfunctional families, of being trapped in an unhappy marriage or in a despised job or career ... Chronic stress comes when a person never sees a way out of a miserable situation. It's the stress of unrelenting demands and pressures for seemingly interminable periods of time. With no hope, the individual gives up searching for solutions.

The worst aspect of chronic stress is that people get used to it. They forget it's there. People are immediately aware of acute stress because it is new; they ignore chronic stress because it is old, familiar, and sometimes, almost comfortable.

Chronic stress kills through suicide, violence, heart attack, stroke, and, perhaps, even cancer. People wear down to a final, fatal breakdown. Because physical and mental resources are depleted through long-term attrition, the symptoms of chronic stress are difficult to treat and may require extended medical as well as behavioral treatment and stress management.

Categories of Stress

Beyond the length of time that stress persists, there are different types of stress. Rather, there are different ways that stress can affect us.

Emotional

This is the stress that influences our ability to focus. When people complain about being stressed out or feeling mentally fatigued, the stressor is likely to be an emotional one.[13] On an individual level, mitigating emotional stress is usually done through relaxation techniques and conversation. However, one can also eliminate emotional stress by separating the individual from the stressor.

Physical

Physical stressors are literally pains in the body. Whether from an injury, chronic illness, or changes in barometric pressure, when the body experiences discomfort it causes stress on the body.[14] Adapting to this stress is possible over time, but unmitigated physical stressors can deplete adaptation energy and become a source of emotional stress.[15]

Chemical

This category covers anything that changes the chemical balance within your body. Obvious examples include stimulants and depressants, but this category also covers unhealthy food or lack of proper hydration.[16] Eliminating stressors associated with these pollutants is not so much an emotional "let's talk it out" process, and may or may not be in the manager's control. Managers may have influence over the unhealthy food or lack of hydration via scheduling water and meal breaks. Adjusting stressors like drugs and alcohol, legal or otherwise, may only be within the manager's purview if job performance or workplace safety is jeopardized. Of course, the detox and routine change itself can become a source of emotional stress.

Stress at Work

The American Institute of Stress reports: that "[n]umerous studies show that job stress is far and away the major source of stress for American adults and that it has escalated progressively over the past few decades." While the factors are numerous, the institute points to workload as the biggest culprit.

Costs

The statistics regarding the financial impact of stress are as numerous as they are staggering. At the time of this writing, workplace stress is estimated to cost organizations 80 billion dollars annually.[17] It starts to make sense when one considers that "[f]orty percent of worker turnover is due to job stress. It costs a company approximately $13,000 to replace the average employee."[18]

In addition, there has been a trend in the last 20 years toward favoring employees in worker's compensation cases pertaining to workplace stress. Increased cost in insurance premiums, while an indirect cost, still represents a cost impact. Health-care costs are almost one and a half times more for employees reporting high stress levels.[19]

Additional stress-related losses can be attributed to absenteeism, diminished productivity, legal costs, insurance expenses, and, unfortunately, accidents.[20]

What Can I Do About It?

Stress stems from three sources: life situations, work, and self.[21] The amplitude of the stress pertains to the balance of stressors with support systems. Workplace managers cannot expect to control an employee's life situations or self, but managers can influence stress at work and counter stressors with more support systems.

Barbara Safani's article "Work Stress: What Are Companies Doing About It?" suggests some potential programs:

- Work–life balance support programs
- Leadership training on worker stress
- Online healthy lifestyle programs
- Onsite fitness centers
- Physical activity programs
- Stress awareness programs
- Financial management classes
- Personal health/lifestyle management coaching

Some readers may look at this list and think: "corporations may have that kind of money, but there's no way my company can afford this stuff." To that I say: everything in live entertainment is adapted from somewhere else, so adapt it! Consider the spirit of these solutions. Make physical activity part of the culture. Encourage self-awareness and communication regarding stressful circumstances.

One of the great aspects of our industry is the diversity of skill sets required to produce it. Take advantage of these skill sets! Here are some examples:

- Even if your company cannot afford to start a series of financial management classes, it may be possible to schedule sessions or lectures with the general manager or chief financial officer.

- Many actors are trained in yoga, tai-chi, Pilates, and other "mind and body" skills. If this is part of the daily routine anyway, why not ask them to invite others in and pass the hat when done?

- Putting a gym onsite may be impractical (space is almost always at a premium), but not every workout requires a rowing machine and Nordic track. A fellow carpenter at the Julliard School used to do pull-ups during lunch break off the theatre's structural steel.

- Two Guys and a Credit Card Productions hired licensed massage therapists for tech periods so that the actors, designers, and staff could reduce physical stress during the process.

Even if an employee declines to take advantage of these programs or strategies, the employee knows the programs are there. It establishes a culture that is serious about stress reduction and may open up an employee to discussion of stressors before burning out.

Sleep

Sleep is commonly one of the first commodities to go when production timelines are constrained. While 24-hour shifts do occur, more often it manifests as a death of a thousand cuts. One night the crew works late and goes from eight hours of sleep to five and a half hours. Then six hours. Then four hours. Suddenly, the sleep schedule is out of whack, all in the name of longer work shifts.

I believe that this is due to a sense of "wasted time" when we sleep. The body is not moving, so it must not be productive time, right? The reality is that asking a crew not to sleep is like asking them to skip a meal or two. There seems to be more time in the schedule, but the time is now less efficient, because the body is less efficient.

This section will lay out the rules of sleep as well as describe some strategies to manipulate sleep cautiously. All-nighters may still be necessary, but at least we can understand how to maximize productivity and what to expect as a consequence.

The Sleep Cycle

Before we can discuss the manipulation of sleep, we should understand how it works. There is a lot of mystery surrounding sleep, but a lot of research as well. According to Helpguide.org, different people need different amounts of sleep. Most require between seven and nine hours, but there are outliers. Furthermore, the same individual may require a different amount of sleep at age 20 versus age 40.

With that many variables, it is important for a manager not to assign stigma to an individual based on sleep needs. A person is not weak or lazy for requiring ten hours of sleep.

According to the National Sleep Foundation, a typical sleep cycle goes through four stages of non-rapid eye movement (NREM) sleep and then into rapid eye movement (REM) sleep.

NREM Stage 1

This is a delicate stage, where the sleeper can easily be roused. Some experience a sense of falling or brief muscle spasms called "hypnic jerks."[22]

NREM Stage 2

This is a period of physical slowdown. The heartbeat slows down as the body relaxes and prepares to move into a deeper sleep. The sleeper is much less responsive to outside stimuli.

NREM Stages 3 and 4

This is when the "deep" or delta sleep begins.[23] The brainwaves slow down, and responsiveness is very low. Once the body goes through these stages, the sleeper is primed to dip into REM sleep.

The National Sleep Foundation also highlights that these stages are the most *physically* restorative.

REM Sleep

This is the stage that is the most *mentally* restorative. The brain processes the day's events and effectively resets for the next day. This is the stage when dreaming occurs.

A full night of sleep represents around five to six complete sleep cycles, from NREM through REM. Think of these stages like a scenic artist's ombre rather than neat little packages. They blend together rather than having hard starts and stops. There is a great article from Harvard Health Publishing called "Repaying Your Sleep

Debt" that goes into this further, and Figure 3.2 summarizes data from that article.

You can see from the chart that the loss of just one hour of sleep is also a loss of some premium REM sleep. That loss needs to be made up to restore optimal functionality.

Sleep Deficit

A savvy freelancer might take what has been written and say: "OK, I need 8.5 hours of sleep per night, and there are seven nights in a week, so I'll frontload the 59.5 hours through the first three days of the week and work the remaining 108.5 hours!"

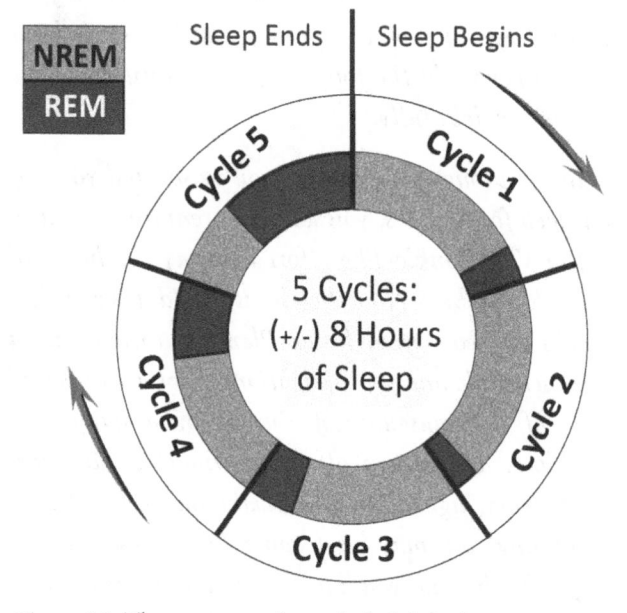

Figure 3.2 The structure of a typical night's sleep.

Think of the overtime ....[24]

Unfortunately, sleep is not a zero-sum game. One cannot add to the "sleep bank" prior to use.[25] There is a cadence to the sleep process, and messing with that cadence means losing sleep and developing sleep debt.

The good news is that there is a limit to how much sleep debt one can accrue. Research suggests that the limit is 20 hours, but that loss can only be paid back in one- to two-hour increments.[26]

Harvard Health Publishing gives the following suggestions regarding how to restore sleep debt:

> *Settle short-term debt. If you missed 10 hours of sleep over the course of a week, add three to four extra sleep hours on the weekend and an extra hour or two per night the following week until you have repaid the debt fully.*

> *Address a long-term debt. If you've shorted yourself on sleep for decades, you won't be required to put in a Rip Van Winkle–like effort to repay the hours of missed slumber. Nonetheless, it could take a few weeks to recoup your losses. Plan a vacation with a light schedule and few obligations – not a whirlwind tour of the museums of Europe or a daughter's wedding. Then, turn off the alarm clock and just sleep every night until you awake naturally. At the beginning, you may be sleeping 12 hours or more a night; by the end, you'll be getting about the amount you regularly need to awake refreshed.*

If a technician explores these options with no improvement, the individual may need help. Sleep apnea, narcolepsy, and various other sleep disorders can seriously hinder a sleep strategy, regardless of how well planned it may be. If a sleep disorder is suspected, consult with a doctor to discuss options.

Circadian Rhythm

Much as humans have an optimal number of work hours, we also have an optimal window of work time. Humans are diurnal creatures, which means we operate best during daylight hours.[27] This is an inherent part of human biology and is unrelated to a personal leaning toward "early bird" or "night owl."

This rhythm is based on a 25-hour day. For those readers who have wondered why it is so easy to stay up late but hard to wake up early, this is why.[28]

How Does Natural Circadian Rhythm Work?

Circadian rhythm has two timekeepers as described by the American College of Emergency Physicians. The first is an endogenous component commonly referred to as an internal clock. Your internal clock, it turns out, is housed in the supra-chiasmic nucleus of the hypothalamus, which makes it really hard to reach in and press the button to adjust for Daylight Saving Time.

Complementing the internal clock, circadian rhythm is also affected by an exogenous component. Basically, this is a combination of all the outside cues that help us determine time. These indicators, called *zeitgebers* (TSYT-ge-buhrs), include eating and drinking patterns, scheduled events, stimulants/depressants, and more. Perhaps the biggest player in circadian rhythm is the light and dark cycle. Makes sense, right? If you see the sun, you are pretty sure it is daytime.

When the Rhythm Is On

If everything is balanced, the start of the work call feels like the start of the day. Wrapping up the work call feels like the end of the day. The technician is focused, alert, and careful about the details of a project. Entertainment professionals usually work with high voltage, heights, fabrication machinery, sharp tools, and even powered vehicles, so this level of functionality is clearly desirable.

While each person is different, as is reflected by early birds and night owls, there are ebbs and flows to circadian rhythm for each individual. Christopher Barnes discusses the best way to take advantage of circadian rhythm efficiency in his article "The Ideal Work Schedule, as Determined by Circadian Rhythms." The highs and lows in productivity during the average workday according to Barnes are shown in Figure 3.3.

As you can see, a "normal" workday would show an increase in focus until it peaks around noon. A decrease follows (which I had always called the "food coma" but is apparently unrelated to food) until about 3:00 p.m. There is a second crescendo until approximately 6:00 p.m., and from there the workday ends.

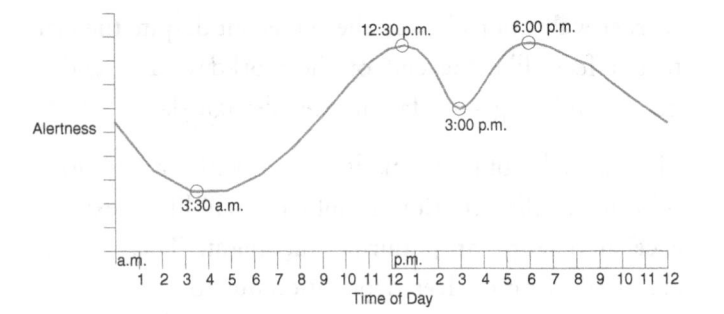

Figure 3.3 Average circadian ebbs and peaks.

Obviously, Barnes is not thinking of tech or show schedules, so it is important to gather data within a given workplace. For those on night schedules, is the 6:00 p.m. time the most productive? Or does the circadian cycle for a 9:00 a.m.–6:00 p.m. schedule translate differently from a 4:00 p.m.–12:00 a.m. schedule, which shows peaks at 7:00 p.m. and slumps at 10:00 p.m.? The key is to pay attention to the details and track productivity.

When the Rhythm Is Off

Many of us experience misaligned endogenous and exogenous factors. This occurs when the body thinks it is one time but the environment says otherwise. Perhaps you have endured a Daylight Savings Time adjustment, or you have travelled a long distance and experienced jet lag. These are common examples.

Consider a technician who works in a theatre with no exposure to outside light. The work call is complete, the worker walks outside, and the sun is out despite the fact that it feels like the end of the workday. The endogenous and exogenous factors are misaligned.

There are a lot of problems associated with a continuous shift in circadian rhythm. Employees will likely experience an energy drop during the night. There is an increased threat of sleep deprivation due to less effective sleep during daytime hours. Circadian rhythm disruption has even been linked to cancer.[29]

So, how does this occur in the entertainment field? Here are some examples:

a) A stagehand works in the scene shop by day but must serve as a deck carpenter on show nights. The performance schedule starts, with shows running Thursday through Saturday nights and a Sunday matinee. While Monday is a day off, the stagehand is expected to work during the day shift on Tuesday and Wednesday. The start of the workday is now regularly changing, and so is the sleep schedule. The stagehand now needs to reset circadian rhythm at minimum twice a week.

b) A freelancer lands a 24-hour gig during fashion week. The work call starts at 8:00 a.m. and ends at 8:00 a.m. the next day. The end is now the beginning, and the circadian rhythm is off.

c) A film crew member goes from a day shoot on Tuesday, to night shoots on Wednesday and Thursday, and back to a day shoot on Friday. Circadian rhythm has shifted twice in half a week. Even with a minimum eight-hour break in between, the body cannot process when it should be sleeping, and so sleep does not occur.

Methods to Overcome the Zeitgeber Conflict

It is widely stated in the medical community that changing circadian rhythm often is detrimental to an employee's health. It will also yield far less productive work and increase the chance of accidents.[30] So, a manager must schedule with care to reduce the risk of accidents and avoid a systemic loss of productivity.

For strategies that mitigate the Zeitgeber Conflict, see "Shift Work" in Chapter 4. Regardless, one should not schedule an employee to work four to seven days' worth of night shifts and then go back to a day or swing shift. This would mean that one would finish a circadian shift just in time to shift again, with no time for recovery.

As a reminder, the human body can adapt to new rhythms if given a chance. Start by changing the zeitgebers. Try to be consistent about when a shower happens, either at the top or at the end of the day. Schedule meals based on the new work schedule. Use blackout curtains if sleeping during day hours, and use electronics and "blue light" sources if staying up at night. The trick is to create cues for your internal clock to adjust to. While there will always be a level of disorientation when a shift starts, adjusting the environment may minimize the linear time of the transition.

Considering Circadian Rhythm

The big takeaway here is that humans are not 100 percent efficient just because we need them to be. Tracking productivity and paying attention to how work is scheduled can yield higher performance. For example, does a lunchbreak scheduled from 11:30 a.m. to 12:30 p.m. rob the team of productive time? Is intensive project work scheduled to start at 3:00 p.m., when productivity is low? Does that have an impact? (see Figure 3.4)

Most importantly, remember that employees who shift from day to night and back again are increasingly at risk for accidents and chronic illness. If possible, minimize the number of transitions to get more productivity and to maximize the safety of the team.

Sleep Deprivation

I once participated in an exhausting conversation where people started to brag about how little sleep they needed to get through the night. This is like bragging about eye

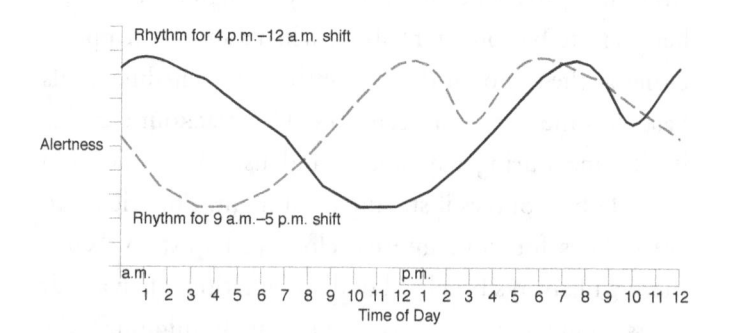

Figure 3.4 Possible night shift ebbs and peaks.

color; it is not really a choice. Worse, it started to pressure the whole team to reduce their amount of sleep to the lowest amount possible. One can see how this might lead to sleep deprivation.

Sleep deprivation is defined as "the condition of being robbed of sleep, in real life or in experiment, as opposed to being unable to sleep."[31] The typical amount of sleep for an adult is between seven and nine hours per night. If an individual gets less than the required amount, sleep deprivation sets in.[32]

A Brief Medical Synopsis

Sleep deprivation is hard to quantify, because there are simply too many variables to consider. Entire medical journals have been written on the findings pertaining to sleep deprivation, and that level of discussion is beyond the scope of this book. That said, ignoring the dangers that sleep deprivation represents would be foolhardy. What follows is the tip of the iceberg when it comes to sleep deprivation and the damage it can do.

Short-Term Impacts

Michael J. Breus, PhD's article "Sleep Habits: More Important Than You Think" does an exceptional job of describing some of the effects that sleep deprivation can have on an individual:

> *Decreased Performance and Alertness: Sleep deprivation induces significant reductions in performance and alertness. Reducing your nighttime sleep by as*

little as one and a half hours for just one night could result in a reduction of daytime alertness by as much as 32 percent.

Memory and Cognitive Impairment: Decreased alertness and excessive daytime sleepiness impair your memory and your cognitive ability – your ability to think and process information.

Stress Relationships: Disruption of a bed partner's sleep due to a sleep disorder may cause significant problems for the relationship (for example, separate bedrooms, conflicts, moodiness, etc.).

Poor Quality of Life: You might, for example, be unable to participate in certain activities that require sustained attention, like going to the movies, seeing your child in a school play, or watching a favorite TV show.

Occupational Injury: Excessive sleepiness also contributes to a greater than twofold higher risk of sustaining an occupational injury.

Automobile Injury: The National Highway Traffic Safety Administration (NHTSA) estimates conservatively that each year drowsy driving is responsible for at least 100,000 automobile crashes, 71,000 injuries, and 1,550 fatalities.

Long-Term Impacts

Dr. Breus goes on to list the following ailments associated with sleep deprivation:

High blood pressure	Heart attack
Heart failure	Stroke
Injury from accidents	Growth retardation
Obesity	Poor quality of life

In addition, obesity can lead to sleep apnea, Type 2 diabetes, immune system deficiency, and infection. Digestive disorders are six times more likely to develop in subjects experiencing sleep loss.[33]

Cognitive Impact

As if the physical risks weren't enough, sleep deprivation has been linked to several cognitive impairments as well.

Tedium Versus Complexity

Studies have established that tedious and repetitive tasks are very susceptible to impairment and loss of efficiency due to sleep loss. Decision-making tasks that require "substantial planning and mental imagery" suffer under sleep loss.[34]

Sleep Loss Versus Alcohol

Studies indicate that reduced sleep can impair drivers as much as alcohol. An individual awake for 17 to 19 hours performed worse than those with a 0.05 percent blood alcohol level.[35] Those awake for 24 hours functioned as if they had a 0.10 percent blood alcohol level.[36]

Getting the Job Done

Now that we are aware of some of the potential risks associated with sleep deprivation, what can be done about it? It can be difficult for an organization to tell employees to get more sleep, because a manager is not likely to follow employees home and tuck them in.

That would be bad.

What an organization can do is establish protocols that accept the reality of sleep deprivation and plan accordingly.

Need a Lift?

Establishing travel protocols in the case of an anticipated long work call is a great way to reduce dangers on the road. Arranging transportation home or to a hotel on the company's dime is a great way to reduce risk.[37]

Nap Time

A 20-minute nap can go a long way to rejuvenate the body. Fire departments now encourage naps before driving home from 24-hour work calls to make sure the firefighter is driving with reduced impairment.[38] Holding a nap period during the day can be helpful as well, but note the importance of having either a 20-minute nap or a 90-minute nap. Waking up within that approximate window of time breaks the deeper NREM stages or REM sleep and will result in sleep inertia, more commonly known as "grogginess."[39]

Pass the Coffee

As a short-term solution, 75 to 150 milligrams of caffeine can help curb the impact of acute sleep loss. Prolonged use will reduce effectiveness as tolerance develops ... and as it is a stimulant, withdrawal symptoms may develop.

Coffee takes about a half hour to kick in. Taking a 20-minute nap immediately after drinking coffee can yield an even stronger sense of alertness.[40]

Project Manage Appropriately

While suffering through sleep deprivation, consider assigning tasks based on interest. A task that the subject deems exciting or fresh and that requires lots of innovation can maintain efficiency despite sleep loss for up to 36 hours.[41] Complex tasks are mostly efficient in the face of sleep loss, provided that the tasks engage the subject intellectually and are "essentially rule-based".[42] Remember to have all the decisions made in advance, and that the plan is clear from the beginning.

Take Care of the Team

Mindfulness of nutrition, exercise, and good sleep patterns is vital to maintaining a healthy body and sleep hygiene.[43] Offer fruit and water instead of donuts and soda. Encourage a workout period during the day. Lead by example. If the crew sees that management really supports a healthy lifestyle, it may inspire change in the culture of the organization.

Be Safe

Do not mess around when it comes to sleep deprivation.

Sleep deprivation causes car accidents.

Sleep deprivation is linked to disease.

Sleep deprivation contributed to the nuclear meltdowns at both Three Mile Island and Chernobyl.

Sleep deprivation is a catalyst for depression and suicide.

Sleep deprivation kills, and is sinister. People who suffer from it experience reduced cognitive self-awareness to the point that they do not recognize sleep deprivation in themselves and so do not understand what a liability they have become.

Managers cannot tell employees how to live outside work, but by raising awareness and nurturing a culture of wellness, managers can save lives.

Works Cited

American Academy of Sleep Medicine. "Sleep Deprivation." *Sleep 2008 Overview*, 2008, aasm.org/sleep-2008-overview/. Accessed 9 April 2013.

American College of Emergency Physicians. "Circadian Rhythms and Shift Work." Policy resource and education paper, 2003.

American Institute of Stress, "Workplace Stress" (survey), *American Institute of Stress*, n.d., www.stress.org/workplace-stress. Accessed 9 April 2013.

"Anatidaephobia is the fear that somewhere in the world, there is a duck watching you." *Factual Facts*, n.d., https://factualfacts.com/anatidaephobia-is-the-fear-that-somewhere-in-the-world-there-is-a-duck-watching-you/. Accessed 2 March 2020.

APA Help Center. "Stress: The Different Kinds of Stress," 2004. *American Psychological Association.* www.synergyeap.org/index_htm_files/different%20kinds%20of%20stress.pdf. Accessed 2 April 2013.

Barnes, Christopher M. "The Ideal Work Schedule, as Determined by Circadian Rhythms." *Harvard Business Review*, 28 January 2015, https://hbr.org/2015/01/the-ideal-work-schedule-as-determined-by-circadian-rhythms. Accessed 26 July 2018.

Breus, Michael J., PhD. "Sleep Habits: More Important Than You Think." *WebMD*, n.d., www.webmd.com/sleep-disorders/features/important-sleep-habits#1. Accessed 9 April 2013.

Bullen Love, Danielle. *Circadian Rhythm Disruption & the Link to Cancer Risk*. Oncology Times, vol. 39, no. 16, 2017, pp. 1–5, journals.lww.com/oncology-times/fulltext/2017/08250/Circa dian_Rhythm_Disruption_the_Link_to_Cancer.2.aspx. Accessed 26 July 2018.

Cline, John, PhD. "The Mysterious Benefits of Deep Sleep." *Psychology World*, 11 October 2010, www.psychologytoday. com/us/blog/sleepless-in-america/201010/the-mysterious-benefits-deep-sleep. Accessed 2 March 2020.

Davis, Jeanie Lerche. "The Toll of Sleep Loss in America," *WebMD*, n.d., www.webmd.com/sleep-disorders/features/ toll-of-sleep-loss-in-america#1. Accessed 9 April 2013.

Elliot, Diane L. and Kerry S. Kuehl. *Effects of Sleep Deprivation on Fire Fighters and EMS Responders*. Portland: Division of Health Promotion & Sports Medicine, Oregon Health & Science University, 2007.

"Eustress vs Distress." *Brock University*, 2010, brocku.ca/health-services/health-education/stress/eustress-distress. Accessed 5 April 2013.

"Flexplace." *Wikipedia*, n.d. Accessed 28 March 2013.

"General Adaptation Syndrome." *Oracle Foundation*, 8 November 2012, library.thinkquest.org/C0123421/gas.htm. Accessed 9 April 2013.

GoodTherapy. "Does Natural Lighting Make Us More Productive?" *GoodTherapy blog*, goodtherapy.org/blog/natural-lighting-increases-productivity-0104112/, 4 January 2012. Accessed 2 April 2013.

Harrison, Yvonne and James A. Horne. "The Impact of Sleep Deprivation on Decision Making: A Review." *Journal of Experimental Psychology: Applied*, vol. 6, no. 3, 2000, pp. 236–249.

Harvard Women's Health Watch. "Repaying Your Sleep Debt: Why Sleep Is Important to Your Health and How to Repair Sleep Deprivation Effects." *Harvard Health Publishing, Harvard Medical School*, 9 May 2018, health.harvard.edu/womens-www. health/repaying-your-sleep-debt. Accessed 31 July 2018.

Helpguide.org. "Sleep Needs: What to Do If You're Not Getting Enough Sleep." n.d., www.helpguide.org/articles/sleep/sleep-needs-get-the-sleep-you-need.htm. Accessed 31 July 2018.

Lauryn, Dr. "Your Out-of-Whack Circadian Rhythm (and 6 Ways to Trick Your Body into Feeling AMAZING)," *dr. lauryn*, n.d., https://drlauryn.com/hormones-metabolism/ circadianrhythms/. Accessed 31 July 2018.

Lisa, Dr. "A Modern Day Juggling Act: Understanding the Types of Stress," n.d., Doctor-Recommended-Stress-Relief.com. Accessed 9 April 2013.

Maxon, Rebecca. "Stress in the Workplace: A Costly Epidemic," 1999, www.fdu.edu/newspubs/magazine/99su/stress/html. Accessed 13 March 2020.

Mr. 4HWD. "Why I Don't Work Over Time (Usually)." *The Four Hour Workday*, 25 February 2014. www.thefourhour workday.com/why-i-dont-work-over-timeusually/. Accessed 18 November 2018.

National Sleep Foundation. "Sleep Cycles: Everything You Need to Know," n.d., http://sleep.org/articles/sleep-cycles-everything-you-need-to-know/. Accessed 31 July 2018.

Ralston, Derek. "How to Pay Back Your Sleep Debt, the Smart Way," *Life Evolver*, 30 July 2008, www.lifeevolver.com/pay-sleep-debt-smart/. Accessed 31 July 2018.

Random House Dictionary. www.dictionary.com.

Scarbrough, Marsha. "Who Needs Sleep?" *Millimeter Magazine*, 1 October 2006.

"Stress Reduction/Mindful Eating," n.d., upstate.edu/stress/work.php. Accessed 9 April 2013.

"The Man Behind the Buzz: Hans Selye," 2011, Doctor-Recommended-Stress-Relief. Accessed 5 April 2013.

Notes

1 (Random House Dictionary)
2 (Maxon)
3 (GoodTherapy)
4 ("Eustress vs Distress")
5 ("Eustress vs Distress")
6 ("Eustress vs Distress")
7 ("General Adaptation Syndrome")
8 ("The Man Behind the Buzz: Hans Selye)
9 ("Flexplace")
10 ("General Adaptation Syndrome")
11 (APA Help Center)
12 Anatidaephobics are those who "believe that somewhere out there, no matter what they are doing, a duck is sitting there waiting and watching." (Factual Facts)
13 (Dr. Lisa)

14 (Dr. Lisa)

15 ("General Adaptation Syndrome")

16 (Dr. Lisa)

17 (American Institute of Stress)

18 (American Institute of Stress)

19 (Dr. Lisa)

20 ("Stress Reduction/Mindful Eating")

21 (Maxon)

22 Not to be confused with "hypnotic jerks," known for making audiences behave poorly while under hypnosis

23 (Cline)

24 Assuming $25/hour, with eight hours of straight time, time-and-a-half until 12 hours, and double time after:
   $(\$25 \times 8) + (\$37.5 \times 4) + (\$50 \times 96.5) = \$5,175$

25 (Ralston)

26 (Ralston)

27 (Elliot and Kuehl)

28 (American College of Emergency Physicians)

29 (Bullen Love)

30 (American College of Emergency Physicians)

31 (Random House Dictionary)

32 (American Academy of Sleep Medicine)

33 (Elliot and Kuehl)

34 (Harrison and Horne)

35 (Davis)

36 (Elliot and Kuehl)

37 (Scarbrough)

38 (Elliot and Kuehl)

39 (American Academy of Sleep Medicine)

40 (American Academy of Sleep Medicine)

41 (Harrison and Horne)

42 (Harrison and Horne)

43 (American Academy of Sleep Medicine)

Chapter 4
Managing the Work

The moment a project begins, a countdown starts: the countdown to opening night. Whether it's a conference opening, a half-time show, or a piece of theatre, live entertainment has a fixed completion time that can rarely be adjusted without incurring a large loss of revenue. For a smooth-running project, the pressure of an immutable deadline can drive a workforce to achieve almost miraculous feats of productivity. A problematic process, however, can suck the life out of a technician.

Addressing the notion of wellness and burnout without first talking about the demands of the industry would be like debating swimming technique without ever getting in the water. Personal wellness alone cannot stave off burnout if a workplace makes unreasonable demands of the employee. I refer to this as scope management, and it is essential to create a productive and healthy work environment.

In this section, we'll discuss how management mechanisms can be used to manage the scope of a project. We'll explore the positive and negative impacts of different tactics used to get more done during a specific time period.

The Triangles of Management

Scope management is all about prioritization and allocation. The prioritization I refer to is less unit based in this instance and more macro level. Questions like "How textured is the detail work for this event?" or "What level of finish are we going for?" are examples of clarification of priority based on aesthetic. "How much of this paint treatment do you need completed before tech?" is an example of clarification based on time. A common shorthand for these prioritizations is a triangle, such as the one shown in Figure 4.1.

"Good" refers to the quality of the product. It meets a lot of aesthetic and practical success criteria and will satisfy everyone on the project. If it's not good, it won't meet all success criteria.

"Fast" refers to linear time. If it's fast, it's a tight timeframe. If it's not fast, there are more hours to commit to completion.

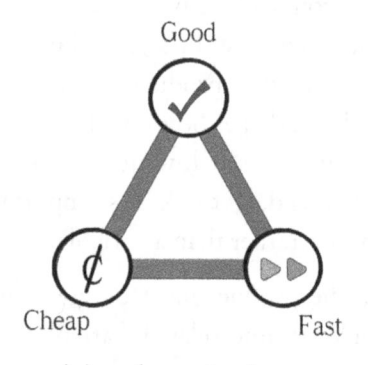

Figure 4.1 The good, fast, cheap triangle.

"Cheap" refers to material and labor costs.

The accompanying expression for the triangle is "Good, fast, or cheap: pick two."[1]

For example, if you want a high-quality product (good) in a tight timeframe (fast), you are likely to spend more on purchasing manufactured items, shipping them quickly, or getting more people hired to get the project completed.

If you want a high-quality product (good) on a tight budget (cheap), you can use fewer people and give them more time to complete the work. You may be able to look around and borrow items or take the time to research vendors and products that are less costly.

If you want it cheap and fast, we can always slap it together, but the product is likely to be less finished (good). Sometimes this has its place, like a last-minute repair mid-show to get through the event (hot glue, anyone?).

Personally, I think it's a bad idea to tell the producer early on that you will deliver a low-quality product, even if it is cheap and fast. First, it all but guarantees dissatisfaction when the product arrives, as everyone expects it to be garbage. Second, the audience doesn't particularly want to see low-quality production elements. To that end, I think it's important to make quality a constant rather than a variable.

So, assuming the product must be good, we look to a second triangle of interrelated variables, indicated in Figure 4.2.

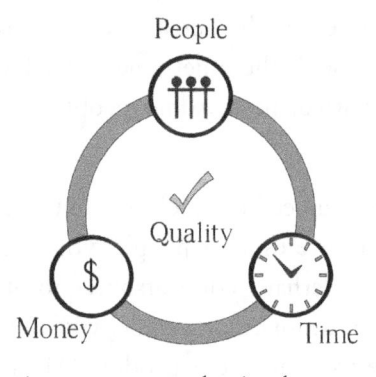

Figure 4.2 The time, money, people triangle.

"Time" refers to linear time. Usually this is measured in hours, but one could consider days, weeks, or even years depending on how compensation is considered.

"Money" refers specifically to materials money.

"People" refers to workers to complete the work.

Again, assuming a high-quality product, I find it helpful to look at which resource is lacking. For example, if you want to achieve a high-quality product, but you don't have a lot of money, you'll need more people and time. Perhaps you have volunteers who are willing to participate, but your schedule has to be flexible, and thus it will take more weekends to complete.

If you don't have many people, you'll need time and money. Perhaps you have one skilled carpenter to build a bunch of furniture. You'll need more time for that person to do all of the work, and you'll probably need to have materials delivered or hire a company to move it all.

In my experience, the most valuable, least available resource is time. If the timeframe is fixed, or the count-down has started, money and people become the big variables.

To be clear, you need not pick two in this circumstance. If you don't have time or people, you can get by with more money. Perhaps you outsource to other shops. If you don't have money or people, you can take a much longer time to complete a product. Most craftsperson art I enjoy fits this category. Suffice it to say, it is hard to get a high-end product with no time, money, or people.

Managing Scope Through Estimation

A technical manager will usually have a budgeting moment. It may happen with spreadsheets and hours of calculation, or it may be an almost instinctive response to a photograph. Regardless of process, somewhere along the way, someone has to decide that a project is producible with the time, money, and people available. This decision results from estimation.

Estimation is really the process of assuming. Some assumptions are items that we have direct control over: assuming the workday is eight hours, that the budget is fixed, or that technical drawings will be completed by a certain date. Other assumptions are based on variables that are outside our control. Perhaps a project is affected by events such as extreme weather events, government shutdowns, or the stock market. Perhaps the labor force changes due to illness or restructuring (Figure 4.3).

Production Variables

In Our Control	Out of Our Control
Prioritization	Creative Team Priorities
Time Usage	Linear Time Available
Staff Allocation	Staff Skills
Order of Operations	Change of Vision

Figure 4.3

Production Expectations

Estimates are the basis of production expectations, and so they are very important. It is my belief that all stress stems from misaligned expectations, and so it is vital to be clear about what the success criteria are and how they will be met.

For example, an electrics crew is tasked with the following success criteria: all front of house and over-stage lighting positions must be hung, cabled, patched, and addressed, and this must be complete by focus. Focus arrives, and the designer walks in to find that all the over-stage positions are complete, and surprisingly, all the practicals are wired and installed, but none of the front of house positions are cabled, patched, or addressed. There is no wasted labor, and the practicals are ahead of schedule, but the designer will likely be upset. They expected a different level of completion by focus, and now they are probably stressed.

My production manager colleague Laura Eckelman[2] once said that she would rather have a technical director deliver less product on time than deliver as much as they can, but late. This speaks to the importance of an accurate assessment of deliverables.

This concept is even more important and formalized in the commercial world. The estimate becomes a bid, which is then the basis for a contract. If deliverables are not achieved on time, it is a breach of contract, and penalties or even legal action may be levied against the company. While contract law is outside the scope of this book, a formal process for change orders (official adjustments to the bid from the client) is highly recommended for organizations to stay solvent.

Estimating Correctly

There are a great many methods for estimation out there. Most of these methods are rooted in assumptions like "You will build this wall in a manner compliant with building code," and so these systems are ineffective for a live entertainment environment.

Good estimates start with clarity of success criteria. Understanding how a particular piece will function, how it will look, and how long it will last is key. This is why complete design packages are so important. It is hard to anticipate the scope of a project if the project is not fully conceived.

Once everyone understands what everything is and how it is supposed to function, one must consider the materials and labor costs for the project. Material estimation is usually quickly achieved through checking prices online or gathering quotes from vendors.

Labor estimation can be more difficult, but there are methods to consider.

Experience-Based Estimation

Understanding how a project will go is easier when one has past experience to draw from. Repetitive exposure to processes will bring some innate understanding. This is why developing a good estimate can be difficult for a manager stepping into a new work environment. There are so many unknowns regarding production capability, it's hard to know what to expect. Checking against previous budgets, conferring with institutional knowledge holders, and relating the projects to similar experiences are all examples of experience estimation.

This estimation technique is well suited to units or projects that are routinely dealt with. For example, if a stock deck is routinely used, and the same method of installation is used, an experience-based estimate will likely suffice.

Critical Path Estimation

This estimation technique involves breaking down the element into multiple steps and assessing how long each step will take.

Consider, for the sake of discussion, the construction of a 2×4 framed platform with a 3/4″ plywood lid. The frame for the unit will be nailed together, and the lid will be attached with 1–5/8″ screws. The estimator considers all the steps in the process, and allocates time and people to them, as shown in Figure 4.4.

Standard Platform Labor

Step	Description	Crew	Hours	Worker Hours
1	Purchase material	1	1	1
2	Cut 2x4 to size	1	0.5	0.5
3	Nail frame together	2	0.5	1
4	Screw lid in place	2	0.5	1
		Linear Time	2.5	
		Billable time	3.5	

Figure 4.4 A critical path for construction of a 4 × 8 platform.

By looking at each individual step in the process, the manager can piece together a total while thinking the process through. This system is well suited to any custom unit but can take more time to create.

PERT Estimation

The PERT system, or Program Evaluation and Review Technique,[3] asks the estimator to consider different production possibilities and then weights them to reduce error. The following descriptions are adapted from the "PERT Estimation Technique" from tutorialspoint. com.

Start with an *optimistic* assessment of each step in the process. The materials all arrive on time, no changes are made to the project, and employees work as efficiently as possible.

Now, develop a *likely* assessment of each step. Maybe there's the occasional mistake, some adjustment or troubleshooting happens, and employees are working at a normal pace.

Lastly, develop a *pessimistic* assessment of each step. It all goes to pot, tons of problems along the way, and the employees aren't working efficiently. (I know many people equate pessimistic scenarios with realistic scenarios, but stick with me on this.)

The estimate for the project is arrived at by applying the following formula to each step:

Step Estimate = (Optimistic Number + (4 × Likely Number) + Pessimistic Number) ÷ 6

Total up all the steps, and you have your weighted estimate number!

It is important to note that there is also a formula for calculating variance in project completion time, which is very important for larger-scale projects, such as theme park installations. The variance equation is as follows:

((Total Pessimistic Numbers) − (Total Optimistic Numbers))^2 ÷ 36

Track the Actual

The expression "practice makes perfect" should be amended to "perfect practice makes perfect." A corollary for this topic would be "perfect tracking makes perfect estimates."

If an estimator works without relating the estimate to reality, the result is that the estimator will get faster at generating inaccurate estimates.

Regardless of what system is used, tracking the actual time spent on a project is the best method to assess the accuracy of the estimate. This can be difficult, as production is often a hectic period. One would also not want to spend so much time tracking that production falls behind.

Short of putting cameras on each employee, my recommendation is to track a project on a daily basis. Consider the platform example from our critical path discussion: rather than having my employee track how long each step took, I would ask for a total amount of time spent on the project during that work call. This could be assessed quickly at the end of the project or the workday, whichever comes first.

To aid tracking at the University of Nevada Las Vegas, the technical directors incorporated an area for recording hours in the drafting title block. The employees tracked build hours right there on the working drawing, and when the drawings were returned, the totals were summed up and compared. While it is true that the level of detail in this assessment is less specific, the result is an accurate point of comparison. This, of course, assumes that employees track correctly and consistently.

If time permits, I also recommend conversation with the people doing the work. The hands-on understanding of the project can yield vital insight and may also encourage employees to work more efficiently, as discussed in Chapter 2 – Motivation.

Allocating Workers

While estimating the number of worker hours accurately is an important step in scope management, the linear time a project will take is greatly impacted by the number of workers involved. An 80-hour project executed by one person working eight-hour days would take ten days to finish. The same project with four people will take a significantly smaller window of time (or it should, at least).

When allocating workers, I think it wise to consider the bare minimum required for a project, and then step up as appropriate. For example, if I were to weld together a 1″ box tube steel frame, I would consider each step along the critical path, as demonstrated in Figure 4.5.

For cold cutting and cleaning the steel, I would assume the steps could be executed by a minimum of one worker. When it comes to grinding and welding, however, I would need at least one more person to maintain fire watch. My minimum number of workers is two, even though one person is doing the work.

Critical Path for Welding Frame				
Step	Description	Crew	Hours	Worker Hours
1	Purchase material	1	1	1
2	Cold Cut 1″ tube	1	1	1
3	Grind tube	2	0.5	1
4	Clean tube	1	0.5	0.5
5	Layout frame	2	0.5	1
6	Weld Frame	2	1	2
7	Fire Watch	1	0.5	0.5

Figure 4.5 A critical path for construction of a metal frame.

Based on these minimums, my worker hour total is 7.5 hours, and the total linear time to accomplish the project is five hours.

It is also important to note that the skill level of the workers has a profound impact on the product. Asking an entry-level worker to execute high-quality structural welds will probably result in it taking longer to complete. This is equally true of taking a career welder and asking them to execute hardwood joinery. Putting talented workers on projects that suit their skill sets primes them for success and yields higher productivity. If productivity is the goal, remember to always put "aces in their places."

Scope Management Through Negotiation

If the scope of a project immediately fits snugly within the limitations of linear time with the material and labor resources available, then it's time to play the lottery, my friend, because you are one lucky duck! I find that, if you try to produce every element to the highest quality possible, the estimate will exceed the allocated budget. This is where negotiations should occur between production and creative to prioritize, adjust, and ultimately bring the project into budget. If scope is not brought within budget, the manager is setting the team up for misaligned expectations and exhaustion.

This may be a controversial notion, but I think it is important to remember that the person with the most power in this negotiation is the area head. Yes, the artistic directors and producers out there have hiring and firing capability, and yes, the production managers are at the top of the production hierarchy. That said, the area head is the one who must say "Yes." There may be consequences, but if the area head says: "This is not doable within the time and money available," then something has to give.

Creatives will do everything in their power to squeeze as much production promise out of a shop as possible. This is their job, so don't be upset when they ask for more than can be delivered. After all, if the creative team knew what it took to build something on budget, they wouldn't need area heads. The area head is the one who assesses the situation and facilitates the negotiation.

If you as the estimator know that the scope is bigger than the time and money allocated, and yet you agree to deliver because you feel pressure from upper management, know that you are in for a rough ride.

Negotiating with Yes, If/ No, But

I find it best to frame negotiation using "yes, if" or "no, but" statements.

"Yes, if," which I credit to Brian Honeycutt at Disney, is an opportunity to have an open-minded dialogue about what the requirements are. It roots the conversation in parameters rather than how the parameters must be met. Consider the following scenarios and examples of "yes, if" responses:

Scenario 1

Request: "Can we get a pair of swords that are stage combat ready for the show?"

Response: "Yes, if you are willing to use what we have in stock, or if you are willing to spend $1,200 to purchase new and have them shipped. As we are underway on the estimate, we could gather the $1,200 by scaling down the finish, by cutting elements A–D, or by asking the producer for more funding."

Often, negotiation will lead to allocation of resources that the area head did not realize were available. Perhaps another department is coming in under budget and can kick some funding over. Perhaps a unit can be substituted by an element from another project. Maybe the company fundraises to get more money. One cannot access these resources without asking.

The "yes, if" technique also works beyond the budgeting phase:

Scenario 2

Request: "Can we hang some extra soft goods in the wings before the day is over?"

Response: "Yes, if we can extend dinner break today by an extra hour. Furthermore, as we do not have staff scheduled to do this, I would need six volunteers."

Even if the team decide they do not wish to alter the schedule or gather the volunteers, the manager has tried to complete the task with the time and resources available.

"No, but," which I credit to intimacy director Claire Warden, is best used when safety is concerned. It clarifies that the discussion cannot go in the direction intended but encourages creative problem solving to get there. Consider the following scenario:

Scenario 3

"I know this is last minute, but can we have our performer jump off the upstage side of our 12-foot tall platform before opening tomorrow?"

A "yes, if" in this scenario might look something like this:

"This would be possible if we acquire the appropriate-sized crash pad ($2,000 new with seven-day delivery time) and build in sufficient training time with stunt oversight. The appropriate stunt coordinator has not been found as of yet, and we need dedicated practice time for the stunt. Given the lack of linear time available, we can add the effect if we acquire the pad, hire a trainer, schedule the stunt rehearsals, and push back opening by a minimum of two weeks."

Now, this answer might be a useful one in an educational environment, as it helps to teach the implications of the request. In the fast-paced world of professional entertainment, however, this answer is unlikely to be seen as helpful.

Let's try a "no, but" instead:

> *"There's not enough time to do this effect safely as described, but we could throw in a stock platform three feet down so it looks like a jump off the back. Does that achieve the same effect?"*

In this case, the answer is no, but the conversation is not over. It acknowledges the value of the request and also moves the team toward an achievable solution that is within scope.

Should the linear time required for a project prove to be higher than estimated, scheduling tools can be used to make up the difference. These tools include overtime, overstaffing, and shift work.

Overtime

Sometimes, a project does not go as estimated. Straight time is defined as "time or number of hours established as standard for a specific work period in a particular industry, usually computed on the basis of a workweek and fixed variously from thirty five to forty hour."[4] For the purposes of this book, overtime will be considered to be any working period outside straight time. For example, a salaried employee who works 60 hours is working 20 hours' overtime, even if there is no remuneration for the extra time.

The use of overtime can impact the health of an employee if scheduled indiscriminately.

Before delving into this issue, it is important to clarify the roots of the information. While there has been investigation of overtime's impact on productivity, there is not as much research as in, say, the negative impact of sleep deprivation. One of the most commonly referenced studies of overtime impact was initiated by the Business Roundtable in 1980.[5] The results of the study generated a curve to suggest the impact of extended use of overtime has on productivity and efficiency.

The study has gaps of information, so there have since been many attempts by subsequent researchers to confirm or deny the results. While it is imperfect, at the time of this writing the majority of researchers have deemed the Business Roundtable results as an accurate measure of productivity in a given timeline.[6]

The work of Sara Robinson will be referenced often in the next section. Sara Robinson is a reporter who extrapolated data from the curve and put it into laymen's terms in her article "Bring Back the 40 Hour Work Week."

Why 40 Hours?

A series of studies run by Frederick W. Taylor and his contemporaries found that the 40-hour work week yields the most equitable balance between input of resources and output of product.[7] For the purposes of this discussion: productivity is a measure of generated product, or project completion, based on the input of resources, or labor.

The study *Impact of Extended Overtime on Construction Labor Productivity*, initiated by Awad S. Hanna, Craig S. Taylor, and Kenneth Sullivan in 2005, compiled data from 500 different contractors in an attempt to qualify the impact of overtime on the productivity of their organizations. Through regression techniques, they were able to extrapolate an equation that predicted how crew scheduling affected labor efficiency to within 15 percent of the actual efficiency rates.[8] The results showed a measurable drop in productivity when overtime hours were worked over several weeks. According to Robinson,

> *industrial workers have eight good, reliable hours a day in them. On average, you will get no more widgets out of a 10-hour day than you do out of an eight hour day. Likewise, the overall output for the work week will be exactly the same at the end of six days as it would be after five days.*

This is primarily due to the onset of physical fatigue in the ninth hour and exhaustion somewhere between the tenth and the 12th hour. This establishes a connection between employee wellness and productivity.

In addition to costs due to lost productivity, overtime for crew can be expensive. In a work environment where an hourly wage is the norm, one can expect to pay a minimum of one and a half times the standard rate for every hour of overtime. Managers are effectively paying a premium for less productive employees due to fatigue.

Technical managers may see how these costs apply to labor-intensive employees, but what of the draftspeople, engineers, and managers who are required to sit at a desk and work? They are often salaried, they are not as physically taxed by their work, and so extra hours from them are often seen as bonus productivity. The reality is that mental fatigue begins to take its toll.

Robinson reports that "knowledge workers," or workers who "think for a living,"[9] have approximately six productive hours in the day. This sheds light on the productivity epidemic of "slacking at work" seen in many corporations at the time of this writing.[10] The impact in a corporate environment is wasted time and money, perhaps due to personal use of company assets or socializing through digital media. Loss of money is bad enough, but in technical theatre, office positions are usually those of higher authority and responsibility, where much of the planning and decision making is done. What is the impact?

Exxon and Morton Thiokol similarly employed high-ranking knowledge workers to make decisions and wield authority: Joseph Hazelwood, who captained the *Valdez* oil tanker, and manager Gerald Mason, who overruled engineers to ensure the launch of the Challenger space shuttle, for example. Through a series of investigations, fatigue of decision makers has been linked to those disasters as well as the meltdowns at Three Mile Island and Chernobyl.[11] Extended overtime wears out skilled personnel and if left unchecked, can cause catastrophic accidents.

If Overtime Is So Bad, Why Do It?

There is an exception where overtime can yield more overall productivity within a linear timetable. According to the Business Roundtable study, moving to a 60- to 70-hour work week for a short window of time can boost results, but there are limits to this practice.

The productivity ratio is not one to one. If a team normally puts in 40 work hours over five days (100 percent time), a manager can expect a baseline of 100 percent productivity. If the crew pushes to 60 work hours over five days (150 percent time), a manager can expect 125–130 percent productivity. Again, this reduction is attributed to fatigue in the ninth hour and the onset of exhaustion somewhere between the tenth and the 12th hour.

Consider the cost analysis when the impact of productivity loss is matched with the premium pay of a 40-hour week versus a 60-hour week. Assume a rate of 25 dollars per hour, an overtime rate of $37.50 after 40 hours, and an overtime productivity percentage of 130 percent.

Straight Time: $(40\,h \times \$25/h)$

$(40\,hours \times (100\% Productivity/100\% Time)$

$(\$800)/(40\,h \times 1) = \$800/40\,h = \textbf{\$25/h}$

Overtime: $((40\,h \times \$25/h) + (20\,h \times \$37.50))$

$(60\,hours \times (130\% Productivity/150\% Time))$

$(\$800 + \$750)/(60\,h \times 0.87) = \$1,550/52\,h = \textbf{\$29.80/h}$

So, overtime drives the overall cost per hour of productivity up by almost 20 percent.

In live entertainment, the necessity of overtime may come from a variety of sources. If material deliveries run late, or the crew works slowly, one could expect a compressed build schedule. Changes from the artistic team can greatly impact the scope of a project.

If those issues hit during the build phase, there is more linear contingency time than if the change develops during the tech rehearsal phase. Thus, a manager may be able to adjust the plan without requiring extra work hours.

During load in or tech, however, when deadlines are imminent, there is less linear time contingency, which may call for more drastic scheduling measures to stay on schedule.

Mitigating the Loss

The Business Roundtable findings suggest that eight 60-hour work weeks are just as productive as eight weeks of 40-hour work weeks. Furthermore, three 80-hour work weeks are just as productive as three 40-hour weeks. If the drop in efficiency plays out further, this suggests that four 80-hour weeks are actually *less* productive than four 40-hour weeks, as shown in Figure 4.6![12]

It is important to emphasize that this study focused on construction and not live entertainment, which is a different industry in many respects. That said, we can at

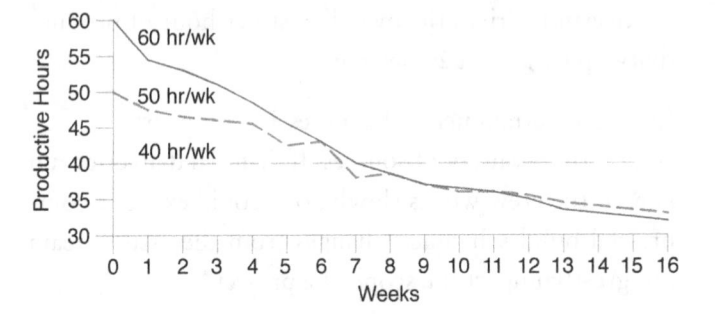

Figure 4.6 Productivity across work weeks.

least accept the possibility that a drop in productivity occurs over weeks of long hours. Perhaps we can also agree that more study on this matter is required.

Accepting the premise of reduced productivity over weeks of long hours, a manager must therefore consider that the longer the period of overtime, the less effective the work will be. Evan Robinson, software engineer, reports that he has seen programmers actually make negative progress by working longer hours. The team would make so many mistakes that the time spent fixing them outweighed the gains.

The message is clear: a productive employee can only effectively work overtime for short windows of time. The longer the hours per day that a manager utilizes, the fewer days a manager can maintain productivity.

Swapping in fresh workers is also a viable solution. If the overtime hours must be maximized over two weeks, one could alternate crews. For example, Crew A works a 60-hour week and then takes a week off. Crew B works 40 hours in week one and then works 60 hours in week two. In theory, a manager could then expect an overall productivity increase of 112–115 per cent for both weeks without a reduction due to exhaustion of Crew A in week two.

Overstaffing

Overstaffing, commonly referred to as "overmanning" in industry parlance, is defined as "to oversupply with [workers] especially for service."[13] This oversupply of staffing is commonly referred to as over hire labor or temporary workers. In theatre, we deal with two kinds of schedule acceleration:

> There are two technical and legal terms associated with schedule compression or acceleration: mandated acceleration and constructive acceleration. Mandated acceleration occurs when the owner requests an earlier completion date than agreed to in the contract. Constructive acceleration occurs when the contract end date stays the same despite a late start, other delays, or an increased scope.[14]

In construction and manufacturing, there are times when a client bumps up a timetable, or there is a shortage of materials from a supplier, or weather causes delays. When this happens, it is common to hire more contractors onto the project to get back on schedule.

For the purposes of the following discussion, overstaffing occurs whenever the average number of crew or staff in a given workplace is exceeded. Whether the need for overstaffing is built into an estimate or initiated in reaction to schedule acceleration, the following considerations apply.

Also note that this section refers to overstaffing within a given department. Having electricians load in while carpenters are onstage, or having one team of carpenters loading in while another team builds elsewhere, represents "task stacking,"[15] the repercussions of which are not in the scope of this book.

Inefficiency

Overstaffing seems like an easy way to offset a deficit of worker hours. One need not worry about the fatigue or exhaustion associated with overtime and shift work, and the work call is much simpler to schedule.[16] In theory, a work-hour need can be met by hiring more straight-time employees to meet the estimated labor. The reality is that there is much potential inefficiency associated with this tactic.

The following description of influencing factors in the construction and sheet metal manufacturing worlds reads as if it referred to technical theatre directly:

> *Some of the problems include inefficiencies due to physical conflict, high density of labor, congestion, and delusion of supervision. Material, tool, and equipment shortages may occur due to the increased number of workers. Due to a greater demand from the architects and engineers, timely responses may not be provided to questions regarding design clarifications. In addition,*

coordination and control become more difficult. The demand for labor may introduce less productive workers. Therefore, supervision that is more intensive is necessary to retain a high level of quality. There are some influencing factors in implementing overmanning. For instance, adequately skilled workers must be available in the market place, and there needs to be enough space in the work area for additional workers.[17]

One can infer from the list of inefficiencies that there is a loss of productivity, but with so many influences, how can a manager quantify the loss?

A study entitled *Impact of Overmanning on Mechanical and Sheet Metal Labor Productivity* by Awad S. Hanna, Chul-Ki Chang, and Jeffrey A. Lackney attempted to do just that.

The researchers deemed it too difficult to account for how much productivity was lost due to each individual inefficiency. There is simply too much variety in work force, manager skill set, and material availability to have a baseline from which to compare. A macro approach yielded a clearer understanding of productivity. By comparing the actual total work hours with the estimated total hours, the researchers eliminated the necessity of analyzing each individual variable. The team developed the following equation to determine the percentage of efficiency lost due to overstaffing:

Percentage loss of efficiency = ((actual total work hours − (estimated work hours + approved change hours))/ actual total work hours) × 100

To put this to use, imagine that a costume shop estimates it will take two staff drapers 20 linear hours to complete a garment. The estimate therefore calls for 40 work hours (two workers × 20 hours = 40 work hours).

Ten linear hours into the build process, some changes are made in rehearsal, and the producer approves the changes. The garment has an extra 30 work hours of labor approved, but there is no more linear time in the process before the garment will be needed. The shop brings on three temporary workers to assist with the garment.

In the end, the garment takes 77 hours to complete. So, putting the equation to use:

((77 actual hours − (40 estimated hours + 30 approved change hours))/77 actual hours) × 100

Working through the equation:

(77 h − 70 h)/77 h = 7/77 × 100 = 9 percent loss

The formula suggests a 9 percent loss in efficiency. However, this percentage is only useful if there is also a gauge of the extent to which overstaffing was utilized. This is often done by calculating the peak personnel power/average personnel power ratio; a ratio greater than one represents an overstaffing situation. Again, consider our costume shop. Two staffers is the average personnel power. The peak personnel power is five (two staffers plus three temporary workers = five).

5 peak manpower/2 average manpower = 2.5 peak over average ratio

For the sake of conservative numbers, the study only considered ratios greater than or equal to 1.6. Figure 4.7 illustrates a consistent result.[18] The larger the number of workers (actual peak personnel power), and the greater the disparity between the normal crew size and the overmanned crew size (peak over average ratio), the greater the percentage of productivity loss (see Figure 4.7).

The graph shows that, regardless of original crew size, the more additional workers put onto a project, the greater the loss of productivity. The graph also suggests that the larger the original crew size, the larger the productivity loss due to overstaffing. In practical terms, the graph suggests that a normal crew of 14 overstaffed to a crew of 50 (or 2.8 peak over average ratio) was 39.2 percent inefficient. This equates to a crew of 50

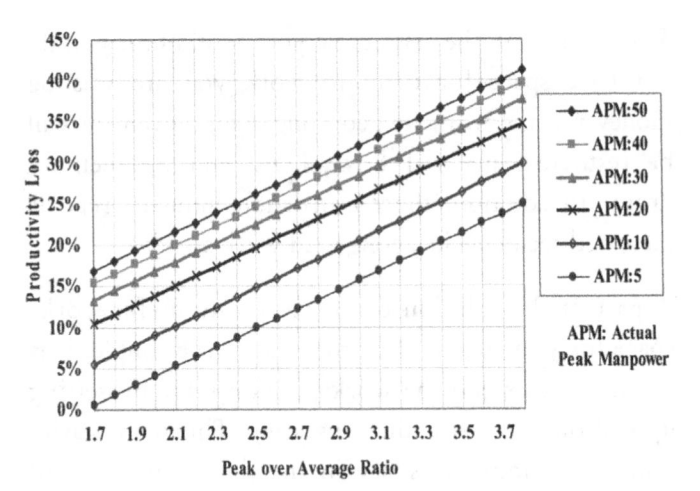

Figure 4.7 Peak over average ratio from impact of overmanning on mechanical and sheet metal labor productivity.

functioning as a theoretical crew of 30 at 100 percent efficiency:[19]

$$(50\ crew) \times (1.0 - 0.392) = (50\ crew) \times 0.608 = 30\ crew$$

This was a study dealing with mechanical and sheet metal laborers, so why should technical theatre managers be interested? Simply put, this same equation could be applied at a manager's shop or theatre to gauge productivity when overstaffing. If one finds inefficiency, one can then attempt to adjust practices to reduce the inefficiency.

Improving Inefficiency

Overstaffing inefficiency is a function of disrupting workflow.[20] There are steps, however, that a manager can take to mitigate this loss of efficiency.

You can hire all the extra crew you want, but if you do not have space for them to work you are wasting money.[21] If the worksite gets congested, movement will be restricted, material flow slows, and productivity drops. In addition, the construction industry reports increased accidents in a congested work area.[22]

A part of the solution can be to create useful workspace for your team. On Broadway, for example, it is common to extend the workspace on stage by setting up scaffolding over audience seating. This temporarily transforms unusable space in the theatre into useful workspace.[23] Similarly, a trap room or lobby space may be utilized.

Consider workflow. Many manufacturers organize their shop layout to reflect the order of operations required to assemble a product. If a design requires lots of soft covered steel flats, the welders assembling frames should not work amidst the carpenters covering the frames. Instead, the welders should be situated so that frames feed to the carpenters' worktables while also isolating the hot work from flammables. When units are finished, flats should be stored by the exit rather than burying other work in progress. This reduces obstructions and traffic in egress paths and keeps workers out of the way of processes that do not involve them. Simple adjustments can go a long way when a large crew is engaged.

It can also be helpful to delegate space based on the needs of the different departments. Look at the order of operations of each process and plan a space schedule based on linear time estimates; for example, installing electrics in the house while sets are being installed onstage during a load in. When loading in, consider traffic patterns of gear and personnel to ensure timely delivery of necessary labor and materials. This will reduce the possibility of departmental miscommunication affecting scheduling or causing accidents. For example, if a temporary worker is told to screw down a deck underneath electricians who are hanging a moving light, it is likely that the worker will not know to ask whether or not the work area is safe.

As crew size increases, more supervision will be required. The additional crew will likely not be intimately aware of the nuances of a project, so they will need more guidance.[24] Whether it is a matter of hiring more supervisors or empowering veteran crew members, delegating leadership to answer questions and allow management to keep an eye on the big picture is vital to ensuring productivity.[25] This is just as much a matter of efficiency as it is a matter of safety, as the heightened conditions may increase project tunnel vision and reduce environmental awareness.

If additional supervisors are hired or assigned, they must be fully briefed on both the project and their responsibilities prior to the crew's arrival. This is especially important when responsibility shifts to a different supervisor.[26] This is common when a scene shop delivers scenery to a house crew, or when multiple departments are involved in a single project. There will likely be an added cost associated with bringing in more supervisors, so the impact of inefficiency must be weighed against the added expense of the additional hire.

The skills of the workforce hired will also impact productivity. When delegating tasks, be sure to consider what individual crew members will be able to achieve effectively, or plan to supervise closely.[27]

Consider training time for the crew. A group of staff employees who are familiar with a space may only need to learn about the needs of the production. A group of new staff who have never worked in the space before will need to fill out paperwork, learn where materials and tools are stored, figure out the language of the environment, and find the bathrooms; factor this time into your estimates. One solution to alleviate these issues is to match up temporary hires with a veteran staff member early on in the process.

Getting a large crew to work efficiently takes time. It is like machining identical parts. The first part takes the longest to jig up and establish order of operations; then the rest move along much more quickly. As an over-staffed crew begins work, the new dynamics of the shop evolve as the crew finds its new groove. If one plans to overstaff for one or two days, it might be wise to avoid establishing new dynamics and consider overtime or shift work as alternatives.

Shift Work

Shift work is defined as "a system of climate where an individual's normal hours of work are, in part, outside of normal day working and may follow a different pattern in consecutive periods of weeks."[28]

Typically, work shifts are broken down into three eight-hour shifts: day, swing, and night. Ten- and 12-hour shifts are also common. Usually, shifts are staffed by different sets of full-time employees. Shift work can be advantageous if one hopes to maintain productivity over a 24-hour period when executing a similar task. Law enforcement, medical, transport, and travel industries all make regular use of shift work.

Technical theatre also makes extensive use of a modified form of shift work. Assuming the production is the employer, different sets of fresh hands are brought in to maximize productivity. Technical managers may refer to shifts as "workday" and "show call" and "late-night turnover." Shift work is a great way to maximize the use of space at a theatre, which is at a premium in both cost and availability during load in or tech periods. One can often find a crew executing notes onstage and then leaving so that a show crew can run rehearsal. Perhaps the paint crew is working the night shift so that they can work undisturbed.

From a productivity point of view, this solution seems to make perfect sense. It maximizes the use of resources over linear time, avoids the expense and inefficiency of extended overtime, and maintains the same level of supervision. Furthermore, when one group of workers passes its eight-hour productivity threshold, a fresh group is brought in. Unfortunately, there are limitations to this labor model.

Circadian Rhythm

As established in Chapter 3, humans have an optimal number of work hours. We also have an optimal window of work time. That work time is heavily influenced by circadian rhythm, which in turn is influenced by our internal clock and external cues to the body regarding time of day. Without these cues, the body would be unable to adjust to Daylight Savings Time or a different season.

The best method to deal with a prolonged night shift is to have a dedicated employee work it full time. It is possible to retrain one's circadian rhythm through a regimented schedule. By blacking out light during the newly established "nighttime" and firmly establishing a sleep schedule, possibly with melatonin supplements, one can hope to adapt in four to seven days.[29] Once on the new schedule, there is no circadian shift.

For shorter stints requiring night shifts, or if a dedicated employee cannot be found, there are two prominent strategies. The first is to use a different employee for every block of night shifts, as shown in Figure 4.8.

For example, if a shop of five staff carpenters must also serve as fire guards for five shows in a season, each carpenter would be assigned one show and work the night shift in a solid block once per season. In this way, each person shifts off and on the diurnal schedule once per year. In optimal circumstances, they would have seven days prior to each transition to ensure a complete circadian shift before working.

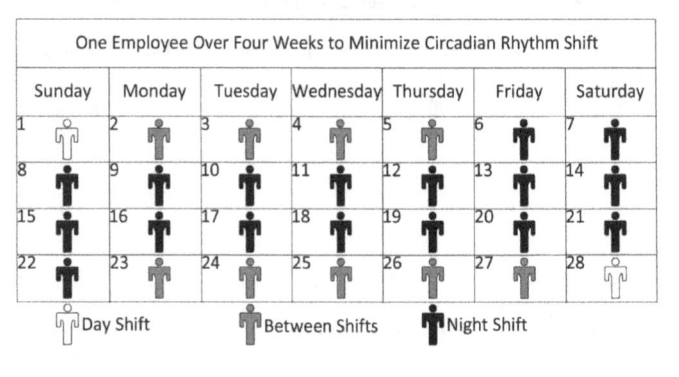

Figure 4.8 Block shifting.

An alternate method, popular in Europe, is to work as few night shifts in a row as possible, as shown in Figure 4.9.

For example, a stagehand works one night shift per week. One night is not enough to shift a circadian rhythm, so if five stagehands rotated the night shift every night, none of them would get off the diurnal schedule. That said, this stagehand will likely have reduced productivity during that window of time.

Once the duration of shift work has been decided, the question remains: how should a manager divide the day? In some cases, there is not much choice. If you only have two employees and you need 24-hour supervision because it is an outdoor event in a public place, 12-hour shifts are your only option. Your best option is to break up the night shift so that each employee has some sleep during the night and some awake time in the day, for example by having the shift change occur at 2 a.m.

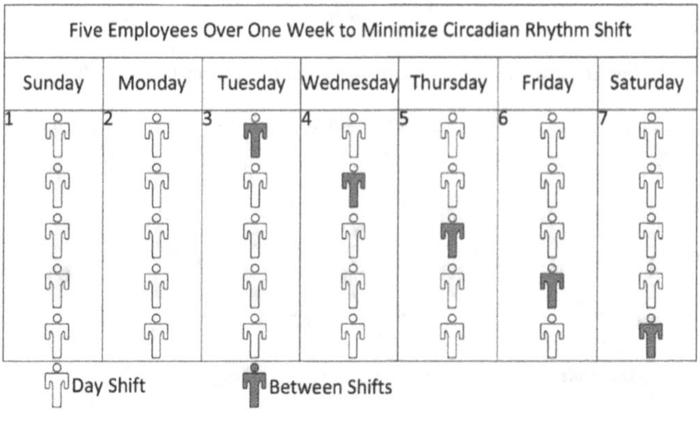

Figure 4.9 One night shifting.

The European model of "one night of night shift" works better with eight-hour shifts. With a minimum of four employees, the most comfortable rotation is: day shift, swing shift, night shift, day off, repeat. This takes advantage of that 25-hour natural rhythm, as an employee has a longer, rather than a shorter, span between start times (see Figure 4.10).

For example, an employee works a day shift starting at 6 a.m. on day one. On day two, the employee switches to a swing shift starting at 2 p.m. That is 32 hours between starts. If that same employee starts a swing shift at 2 p.m. on day one and then a day shift starting at 6 a.m. on day two, there are a mere 16 hours between starts.

There are other strategies that have proven successful in industry. A manager could reduce the length of the night shift and increase the length of the day shift. It is possible to overlap reduced night shifts to disperse the burden and minimize the impact on an individual. In the case of drafting or customer service, one could make use of flexplace and use employees on a different circadian rhythm due to time zone differences. For more on flexplace, see Chapter 2.

One Employee Over Four Weeks to Minimize Circadian Rhythm Shift						
Sunday	Monday	Tuesday	Wednesday	Thursday	Friday	Saturday
1	2	3	4 Off	5	6	7

Day Shift   Swing Shift   Night Shift

Figure 4.10 One night of one shift in action.

Health Concerns

Shift work can become a health hazard if handled poorly. Prolonged abuse of circadian rhythm can lead to sleep deficit, sleep disorder, sleep deprivation, sleep apnea, obesity, diabetes, and cancer.[30]

Technicians are often called in to work hours reserved for the night shift. Perhaps the sound team works late to set levels undisturbed, or a paint crew comes in for late-night paint notes. These technicians may then attempt to drive home. This requires them to use the "tracking" function of the brain, which is also the function most hindered by a lack of sleep.[31]

As we recall from Chapter 3, sleep deprivation carries many health hazards with it. Consider the dangers when scheduling shift work, and do not let your employees drive home when exhausted.

Works Cited

Alagarsamy, Karthick. "Impact of Construction Schedule Compression," Department of Civil Engineering, Auburn University.

Cardone, Elisa, Production Supervisor. *DRAM149: Production Planning Course.* 2013.

Conner, Cheryl. "Employees Really Do Waste Time at Work," *Forbes*, 7 July 2012, www.forbes.com/sites/cherylsnappconner/2012/07/17/employees-really-do-waste-time-at-work/#29fec14b5e6d. Accessed 5 March 2013.

Elliot, Diane L. and Kerry S. Kuehl. "Effects of Sleep Deprivation on Fire Fighters and EMS Responders," Portland: Division of Health Promotion & Sports Medicine, Oregon Health & Science University, 2007.

Hanna, Awad S., Craig S. Taylor and Kenneth T. Sullivan. "Impact of Extended Overtime on Construction Labor Productivity." *Journal of Construction Engineering and Management*, vol. 131, no. 6, 2005, pp. 734–739.

Hanna, Awad S., Chul-Ki Chang and Jeffrey A. Lackney. "Impact of Overmanning on Mechanical and Sheet Metal Labor Productivity." *Journal of Construction Engineering and Management* vol. 133, no. 1, 2007, pp. 22–28.

"Knowledge Worker," *Wikipedia*, n.d. Accessed 3 February 2019.

Lauryn, Dr. "Your Out-of-Whack Circadian Rhythm (and 6 Ways to Trick Your Body into Feeling AMAZING)," *dr. lauryn*, n.d., https://drlauryn.com/hormones-metabolism/circadianrhythms/. Accessed 31 July 2018.

"PERT Estimation Technique," *Tutorials Point*, n.d. Accessed 30 January 2019.

Random House Dictionary. www.dictionary.com. n.d.

Robinson, Sara. "Bring Back the 40-Hour Work Week." *Salon*, 14 March 2012, www.salon.com/2012/03/14/bring_back_the_40_hour_work_week/. Accessed 4 March 2013.

Sammler, Bronislaw, Production Supervisor. *DRAM149: Production Planning Course.* 2010.

The Business Roundtable. "Scheduled Overtime Effect on Construction Projects." A Construction Industry Cost Effectiveness Task Force Report, 1980.

Thomas, H. R. "Effects of Scheduled Overtime on Labor Productivity." *Journal of Construction Engineering and Management*, vol. 118, no. 1, 1992, pp. 60–76.

Thomas, Randolph and Raynar, Karl. "Scheduled Overtime and Labor Productivity: Quantitative Analysis." *Journal of Construction Engineering and Management*, vol. 123, no. 2, 1997.

Notes

1 It is possible to provide product that is good, fast, and cheap, but only if the success criteria are flexible. Improv shows, dance pieces, devised work, and other extremely flexible projects are examples of this.

2 Nicknamed "Nemesis."

3 (PERT Estimation Technique)

4 (Random House Dictionary)

5 (The Business Roundtable)

6 (Thomas, H. R.)

7 (Robinson)

8 The study applied only to union and general contractors specializing in "labor-intensive work."

9 ("Knowledge Worker")

10 (Conner)

11 (Robinson)

12 The Business Roundtable Curve of productivity is confirmed in the 1997 study "Scheduled Overtime and Labor Productivity: Quantitative Analysis" (Thomas and Raynar)

13 (Random House Dictionary)

14 (Hanna, Chang and Lackney)

15 (Hanna, Chang and Lackney)

16 (Hanna, Chang and Lackney)

17 (Hanna, Chang and Lackney)

18 (Hanna, Chang and Lackney)

19 Note: This equation only applies when overstaffing is used for a significant portion of the process. Using the equation to calculate lost efficiency when overstaffing is utilized for a single day on a three-month project will not generate an accurate estimate.

20 (Alagarsamy)

21 (Sammler)

22 (Alagarsamy)

23 (Cardone)

24 (Alagarsamy)

25 (Alagarsamy)

26 (Alagarsamy)

27 (Hanna, Chang and Lackney)

28 (Random House Dictionary)

29 (Dr. Lauryn)

30 (Elliot and Kuehl)

31 (Elliot and Kuehl)

Chapter 5
Case Studies

So far, we have isolated several strategies developed by other industries to increase the productivity of employees. You may be wondering how these strategies have been applied to the entertainment industry.

What follows is a series of real-life examples of organizations that have wrestled with the challenges of employee productivity, and what strategies and tactics they used to maximize efficiency.

Through interviews and email conversations held in 2013, professionals from VHC Inc., Syracuse Stage, J&M Special Effects, and Cirque du Soleil's *Iris* will share their experiences with schedule compression, employee retention, and employee health considerations. These interviews originally contributed to the thesis *Increasing Productivity Through Employee Wellness*.

In addition, through a phone interview in 2019, we will learn about the implementation of wellness initiatives at the Tony Award-winning Utah Shakespeare Festival.

Please note that all case studies will be discussed in the past tense. This is not meant to imply that organizations do or do not continue to follow these practices, but simply to reflect the accuracy of the information at the time of the interview.

VHC Inc.

VHC Inc. is a shop out of St. Paul, Minnesota specializing in audio and lighting equipment for industrial events. They work on anything from 100-person ballroom meetings to 20,000-person concerts, with budgets between $35,000 and $500,000.

The person I spoke with chose to remain anonymous, and to honor their wishes, I will use the pseudonym "Taylor" and the gender-neutral pronoun "they/them."

Taylor was employed at VHC Inc. as a salaried staff member for the audio department. Taylor would function as management, labor, and show support. They were involved in planning the system, prepping the pack, travelling to the site of the event, leading crew at load in, technical rehearsing, running, and striking the event. Over the course of a given production, Taylor would run varied crews, coordinate with other departments for the load in process, and function as the head of their department for a given project.

VHC typically booked gigs well in advance, which meant there was ample time to pull, test, and prep equipment for the events they were contracted for.

Load in, however, was another story.

The businesses that hired VHC also rented the venues for the events. In an attempt to keep costs down, these clients attempted to complete the event within the shortest possible rental period. To the clients, it was more cost effective to pay VHC a few tens of thousands of dollars more for overtime than to extend the rental and pay the venue a few hundreds of thousands of dollars.

A typical schedule for the crew chief and the crew would unfold as follows:

Day 1: 8 a.m.–6 p.m. Load in (ten hours)
Day 2: 8 a.m.–10 p.m. Tech (14 hours)
Day 3: 6 a.m.–4 p.m. Performances, 4 p.m.–10 p.m. Strike (16 hours)

An atypical schedule could go for seven days, 16 hours a day. On these larger projects, Taylor reported that there were instances of leaving at 2:30 a.m. and clocking back in at 7 a.m.

In addition, it was commonplace for the CEO of a multinational corporation to walk up to a crew chief and threaten never to hire VHC again if the event failed to go smoothly. The VHC competitive advantage of a sterling reputation grew or faltered with each project. Taylor said that they would develop stress boils on their upper body after double or triple checking the system the night before an event. They also admitted that they could not fall asleep at night because they were so stressed about how the event would go.

Despite the high stress of event execution, VHC Inc. did not experience a lot of turnover. Most of the staff had been there for 20 years or more. Furthermore, Taylor described the company itself as a calm environment with great people. So how did VHC retain its employees and maintain this positive attitude?

It started with the fundamentals. Though salaried and thus exempt from time-and-a-half overtime rates, the team were paid very well. They had a reimbursement system for health insurance, profit sharing after two years, and two weeks of paid vacation per year complemented by generous amounts of paid personal time.

Taylor described a sense of pride in the company itself as the primary motivator. The company held a reputation as one of the best shops for its type of service in all of Minnesota. The shop was kept immaculate. The load in strategies were thorough and meticulous. The facility was in great shape, and they owned and maintained top-notch gear. The additional benefit of profit sharing meant that the employees' retirement bonus was directly linked to how well the company profited in a given year. This encouraged the team to work harder and ensure bigger profits.

Most importantly, Taylor discussed some strategies the organization used to maintain the mental and physical well-being of the workforce. Instead of overtime pay, the team were given paid time off. So, after an 80-hour week on the job, the next week would be a full week off. This allowed the staff to crash for a few days and equalize before heading back to work. Also, if a prep process was particularly grueling, a staff member could take a paid day off to recuperate at any time. There was no stigma attached to this in the office; in fact, it was celebrated. Management believed that voicing a need to clear one's head was a perfect cue to allocate time off. The exception was the event weeks. As long as the staff made those gigs happen flawlessly, they were given wide latitude in their time off.

Taylor also reported that they felt their time and their home life were respected. If Taylor got their work done early, management did not force them to stay. One could expect to show up at 10 a.m. and leave at 1 p.m. during a slow period and still be paid for a full day of work. Taylor fondly recalled a time when the team showed up at 10 a.m. and then all left to go golfing together. In addition, one could request unpaid time off without repercussion as long as it was during a slow period. Taylor once took a month off and travelled internationally. These flex time options sent a clear message from management: do your best work when required, but do whatever you need to do to avoid burnout.

VHC Inc. needed to accomplish a great deal in a tight window of time. VHC made judicious use of hours outside straight time to maximize the amount of work completed within the linear time of load in week. After completion, it took its assets offline to recuperate, ensuring maximum productivity for the next event. VHC also did all the complex thinking and planning prior to the big push, so that fresh minds could complete as much knowledge work as possible. It seemed that it was aware of the impact of sleep deprivation on cognitive thinking. It should also be noted that when it asked sleep-deprived individuals to work, the tasks were physical and varied rather than tedious and repetitive.

VHC had also worked very hard to cultivate pride and loyalty in its workers, even going as far as encouraging the employees to make a personal investment in the organization's financial well-being. The result: most staff stayed for 20 years or more. Taylor left because they were tired of Minnesota and wanted more responsibility. In the interview, they always characterized the stress associated with the job as client generated. Taylor had nothing but good things to say about VHC Inc. and its management.

Syracuse Stage

Syracuse Stage is a LORT C theatre located in Syracuse, New York on the campus of Syracuse University. Its main stage, the Archbold Theatre, has a seating capacity of 499 seats, and its second stage, the Storch Theatre, seats 250.

At the time of the interview, Syracuse Stage produced seven main stage performances from September to June, with scenic budgets ranging from $3,000 to $25,000. It also produced five main stage productions for the Syracuse University Drama department, whose scenic budgets ranged from $2,000 to $5,000.

Randy Steffen served as technical director at Syracuse Stage. Randy handled hiring for his department, approved all technical designs, established work schedules, and coordinated labor. Randy was also a proud father of six children.

Randy's approach to employee wellness started with scheduling. Randy believed that regional theatre must start with a 40-hour work week assumption. At Syracuse Stage, a typical week consisted of four ten-hour days starting at 7:00 a.m. and ending at 5:00 p.m. As technical director, he strove to maintain this work schedule through managing the expectations of the artistic team. By managing the expectations of the director and designers, Randy felt that a technical manager could maintain a high standard of excellence in production.

Syracuse Stage occasionally made use of overtime. Overtime was a logical answer for that organization (as opposed to overstaffing) because the skilled labor pool in Syracuse, New York was fairly small. Some overtime need was anticipated and worked into the budget based on the seasonal calendar. Changeovers at Syracuse Stage could be particularly tight, so the production team often expected some overtime for those as well. During tech/preview, Randy anticipated a 70-hour work week.

Sometimes, however, plans simply went awry. Maybe the design changed in the rehearsal room, or a problem was found during the build process. Whatever the cause, a choice had to be made: develop an alternate solution or buckle down and do the extra work.

The decision to use overtime was greatly influenced by lead time. Randy would have preferred to maximize work time by splitting crews. For example, in the case of a tight changeover, Randy would bring in one crew to strike until midnight and another to start at 7:00 a.m. However, he did not have enough employees at his disposal to do this. Instead, he tried to influence the season calendar.

Usually, Sunday was a day off for the staff, and a show would close on Sunday night. Changeover then initiated on Monday. For tight changeovers, Randy would advocate closing a show with a Sunday matinee. This bought some time on Sunday to get started before getting underway on Monday.

As a guideline, Randy tried to give employees as much down time as they had work time. If there was a 12-hour call, the crew got 12 hours off. There were rare instances of "striking until late then coming in early" at Syracuse Stage, but Randy strove to avoid this practice. He had found a diminishing return, as this schedule "puts tired people in tough places."

If, however, there was a minimal amount of time to complete the changeover, the theatre had to make some hard choices.

For one, upper management had to be notified and then agree to finance more labor. Once approval was given, the technical director approached the crew. If the need for overtime was communicated one week in advance of the need, the overtime work calls were mandatory. If the need was communicated less than a week in advance, and the staff member had a prior commitment, the work calls were optional. In those instances, Randy could usually anticipate that at least half his staff would work the call.

If an estimate suggested extensive use of overtime, Randy would not move the plan forward. He believed that one or two consecutive 50-hour work weeks was an effective way to make up a labor shortfall. However, after the first couple of weeks of overtime, he saw diminishing returns in productivity; so much so that the work accomplished in a 50-hour week was not much more than in a 40-hour week.

The history of technical production lies in the apprentice–master relationship. Randy believed that the roots of that relationship still influence hiring practices today. At Syracuse Stage, compensation depended on responsibility. As technical director, Randy enjoyed vacation time, good benefits, teaching opportunities, and professional development through Syracuse University.

The staff positions beneath the technical director paid significantly less. Because of this, Syracuse Stage brought in recent undergrads with one or two years' experience and expected changeover every two to three years. Randy described the shop as a great place to start a career in technical theatre, which meant that he tried to be upfront regarding compensation and employee expectations during the hiring process.

Randy made use of the 40-hour week for his labor-based crew. He used overtime sparingly, and rarely for more than a week or two at a time. With few exceptions, work calls occurred during daylight hours.

Syracuse Stage retained Randy by addressing his needs. His health-care benefits became more valuable as his family grew, and the down time during the summer allowed recovery time from the season. To retain his employees, Randy empowered them with choice whenever possible. Time off was allocated after difficult weeks, and Randy was upfront about what career development staff could expect at Syracuse Stage. Randy was also very specific during the hiring process to make sure that potential employees were clear about how Syracuse Stage could support them. Randy also attempted to secure new hires who would readily acclimate to the culture of Syracuse Stage.

It should be noted that the crew worked Monday through Thursday, but Randy and his assistant worked Monday through Friday. The lack of crew on Friday allowed more uninterrupted planning and drafting time.

There were rare instances of an employee's work–life balance spinning out of control. Randy offered the following advice to anyone who may have to deal with this issue. Randy believed that the best a manager can do is encourage good practices in the workforce culture and express problems based on job requirements. Because a manager cannot tell an employee how to live, a work–life imbalance must be dealt with through those job requirements.

For example, if a manager suspects that a staff or crew number has come in to work hung over, the manager should address the tardiness and not voice suspicions. If a crew member shows up drunk, it is the manager's responsibility to send that individual home, but be careful: many lawsuits and allegations of workplace discrimination stem from poorly handled conflict. Document all interactions that may lead to dismissal, and make sure to communicate with your supervisor. Expressing concerns one-on-one with the employee can increase the risk of hearsay and miscommunication, so consider having a superior present during such a meeting.

J&M Special Effects

J&M Special Effects is located in Brooklyn, New York about 20 minutes outside Manhattan. J&M provides a wide array of special effects services including, but not limited to, firearms, magic tricks, blood effects, smoke and fog, and pyrotechnic effects. Clients include some of the biggest names from the theatre, television, film, and industrial industries.

At the time of this writing, Bohdan Bushell was a staff production coordinator and pyro technician for J&M Special Effects. Bohdan attributed J&M Special Effects' success to its adaptability to client circumstances and its reputation for safe and professional execution of effects.

Rather than create a single policy that ineffectively accommodates varied industries, J&M Special Effects mimicked the norms of the industry it was working in on a given day.

For theatre, J&M Special Effects employees looked to IATSE Local 1 union rules. They penalized working past five days with the premium rate. They anticipated two five-hour calls with a four-hour gap in between. This meant compensation for ten hours but being around the theatre for 14. They expected an eight-hour turnaround between calls, so if they finished at midnight, they expected to be in at 8:00 a.m. Nonunion theatre was a little less stringent, so the standard ten-hour day became a 12- to 14-hour day.

For film, the standard call was ten hours, but it could be 11 if there was an unpaid lunch break. J&M Special Effects has learned to expect a lot of work on location. Employees brought lots of expendables and equipment with them to create a palette of options from which they could adjust or scale an effect based on artistic needs.

Photo shoots were more hectic. Food was put out all day, but there was never an official break. One simply ate when one could and reacted to the needs of the creative team. The pay scale was based on a day rate as opposed to an hourly rate.

Special events, as with VHC Inc., would usually go from 8:00 a.m. to 2:00 a.m. the next day.

Adapting to the various schedules was not as simple as assigning a pyro technician for the entire work call. The job involved explosives and flammables, so the work required special attention. Bohdan warned of the risks associated with a sleep-deprived operator hitting the go button for an effect that could potentially engulf an actor in flame.

J&M Special Effects empowered employees and gave them a lot of leeway. The technician on site had flexibility regarding how much work could get done based on comfort level. If too tired to proceed, employees would often bill the client for a hotel room. If work must continue, J&M might send out a relief technician to continue the process.

J&M Special Effects would also hold an internal dialogue among its staff to ensure that no one was overtaxed. It was common for technicians to say: "I cannot take that job, it's too soon after the other job." Staff were responsible for the safety of their clients, so J&M Special Effects took staff input very seriously. Generally speaking, everyone wanted the technician to work within a reasonable window of time. Clients that did not respect these parameters did not get effects.

J&M Special Effects enjoyed a certain amount of leverage when it came to client dealings. First, J&M Special Effects was licensed, so clients needed it to enact effects legally. Second, this was a highly desired skill set. The constant demand for special effects kept the company very busy. As reference, there were thousands of stagehands in New York, but merely hundreds of special effects technicians.

The fact that J&M Special Effects is a nonunion organization actually helped it to set the rules. By not being connected to a formal collective bargaining agreement, it could adapt specific work rules to common sense and individual situations. Bohdan gave an example of a well-intentioned rule established in the collective bargaining agreements of the television industry that didn't quite work.

The collective bargaining agreement called for a ten-hour turnaround after a work call. One would naturally think that this means a 14-hour workday would be followed by a ten-hour turnaround window. But if the work call went long, say 16 hours, the ten-hour mandatory turnaround time actually pushed back the call time the next day. This meant if you started at 7 a.m. on Monday and pulled 16-hour days through Saturday, your start time for Saturday was 7 p.m. Under these circumstances, there is no adaptation to circadian shift. By the time the crew made it to Friday, many people had no idea what day it was. This was so prevalent that the industry term "Fraterday" (a conflation of Friday and Saturday) was used for a call that starts in one day and ends in another. No one liked to work Fraterday.

To develop its own rules, J&M Special Effects studied what other industries established as guidelines. New truck driving rules established ten continuous hours off for truck drivers between driving shifts. This was opposed to the old rules, which allowed ten hours off in five-hour increments.

J&M Special Effects took cues from ironworkers. In that industry, there were financial incentives to encourage workers to go out on iron beams in horrible weather conditions, but there was no rule that mandated that an iron worker *must* work in those conditions. It was entirely up to the worker to decide whether or not to go out on the beam, and there was no work-related penalty for opting not to.

Bohdan cited the nonsensical rules that allowed light rail driver Robert M. Sanchez to work a block of time during rush-hour and then get a break until the next block of time during rush-hour. When looking at Sanchez's schedule, one could see that he could never get a sensible amount of continuous time off. In September 2008, Sanchez blew through a stop signal and crashed into an oncoming train, killing 24, including himself.[1] The lessons of these industries allowed J&M to apply sensible rules to the best of its ability.

When it came to enforcing its rules, J&M had some solid sanctions. The first stick, as Bohdan called it, was financial. Once a technician went beyond the standard workday, they needed time off to recuperate. Time-and-a-half was paid from the 11h through the 12th hour, and double time was paid beginning with the 13th hour. With a base rate of $75 per hour for a lead, that could become pretty cost prohibitive, which was the goal. It was in the company's best interest to ensure that enforcement of work rules would hit the producer in the wallet.

The second stick was moral persuasion. This basically encompassed a firm diplomacy in the client–vendor relationship. They would begin a conversation with a discussion of the company's work rules and the client's work rules and see where conflicts arose. Clients often tried to establish a camaraderie or friendship and use it to leverage for accommodations. J&M Special Effects made it very clear that business was not about friendship; it was about paying for services. Having enough distance to say no was imperative to the safety of all involved.

The third stick was the most potent: the law. A pyro technician's license was much like an engineer's license. If something goes wrong with a building, the engineer is personally responsible and will have to answer to the Authority Having Jurisdiction. There were very strict rules regarding transport of explosives and flammables. J&M Special Effects had no interest in bending the rules to save a client a few bucks here and there.

Bohdan's recounting drives home the notion of managing expectations. Adapting to a client's needs is not a matter of caving to a client's every whim. It is a matter of explaining the financial or legal repercussions of a certain choice and allowing the client to make the call as to whether or not to proceed. J&M Special Effects fully supported the health of its employees by empowering them to make decisions regarding scheduling and safety. It is clear that J&M Special Effects was constantly looking to improve its safety practices. By discussing best practices with clients, J&M also raised awareness of how to safely execute potentially dangerous effects.

Cirque du Soleil: Iris

In 2008, Cirque du Soleil (henceforth referred to as "Cirque") was developing a production to honor the world of cinema. The show was built to go into the Kodak Theatre, now the Dolby Theatre, in Hollywood, CA.

The Cirque process had three distinct phases: project, production, and operations. The project phase was focused on adapting the venue infrastructure to suit Cirque's production needs. The project phase would then overlap with the production phase, which focused on building the show. This was a largely artistic and creative development process, and translates to the rehearsal and build phase in a regional theatre model. It also included months of technical rehearsal and fine tuning the show. The production phase then overlapped with the operations phase. The operations phase was devoted to developing a sustainable system to maintain a high-quality show for an extended run.

The technical aspects of the operations phase began in 2010 and marked the transition out of the production phase. To give a sense of timetable, previews for *Iris* were slated to begin in July 2011, and the show was to open on September 2011. In addition, every February the show was to be struck and stored so that the Academy Awards could take place in the venue. Then in March, after the Award Ceremony, the Academy's set would be struck and *Iris* would come back out of storage and set up for the run until the following February.

The technical management team was not under a collective bargaining agreement (CBA). Department heads, while management, were under the CBA, as was everyone else down the hierarchy. CBA employees were divided into two categories: full-time employees and on-call employees. The primary difference between the two categories was that full-time employees were guaranteed 40 hours of work per week.

Much of the scheduling for crew was dictated by the CBA in effect for the theatre. The focus of this study will be on technical management's schedules and special considerations for an extended-run work schedule.

Cirque's expectations for technical management were to maintain high production values and deal with any issues that might come up with operations. Managers were encouraged to reach out for help if the workload exceeded a reasonable workweek.

Cirque also fostered a sense of teamwork and collaboration to ensure technical managers were not facing challenges on their own. Managers worked together to coordinate how they would take their days off; they would cover for each other so that there was never a lack of management in the venue.

It is also worth noting that Cirque encouraged employees to take time off as needed, but a vacation request would need to be filed at least two weeks in advance. This gave management time to adjust schedules and make sure that all tracks were covered for the week of an employee's absence.

The operations phase was very distinct from "creation" when overlapping the production phase. Creation is marked with longer hours and potential frustration, but also with frequent moments of accomplishment in creativity and ingenuity. Those moments of innovation could help motivate employees who might be tired to remain engaged.

The operations phase, however, had more to do with high-quality reproduction of process. So, how did Cirque motivate its employees and keep them fresh and engaged with a potentially repetitive process?

Cirque empowered employees to take time off as needed during the operations phase. This allowed a crew that might have been dealing with high–skill level stunts and effects to stay fresh and focused. In addition, Cirque fostered a sense of community on several levels. On a show level, it built camaraderie with nonmandatory group events: for example, periodic company-sponsored gatherings away from the theatre or a barbeque between performances on a double show day.

On a city level, Cirque developed a sense of involvement through exposure to art. There was a program that allowed staff to attend local artistic and cultural events and then get reimbursed for the cost.[2] Finally, Cirque promoted a sense of wholeness within the organization at large. For example, the cast and crew of *Iris* were offered a trip to Las Vegas, Nevada to meet with crews from the other Cirque du Soleil productions in that town. Crews from different productions would discuss new technology. This strategy was a great way to promote an institutional knowledge in an organic and free-flowing manner.

Cirque's policies reflected the culture of the organization rather than dictating it. The desire to learn and perfect was part of the fabric of the organization, and special events encouraged those values. Guest speakers would periodically contribute at company meetings. The organization would train employees, full time or on call, in safety and pertinent skills to support careers in their focus and periodically across different jobs in the organization. The sense that Cirque supported employee life fulfillment went a long way toward enriching the company through productivity and efficiency.

For managers stepping into this kind of role, it is common to become self-sacrificing. There are many managers who would rather put in an extra 20 or 30 hours a week to make sure the show runs smoothly and the crew works a straight week. This integrity and eagerness to do a good job can keep managers from seeing the big picture.

Some found that, during times of difficulty, walking away to take a break helped to foster new perspective upon return. Or, in other words, an employee might support the production by doing things away from the production. This is not meant to imply that managers always maintained a work–life balance while working *Iris*, but there was an element of choice in some instances.

The idea that a grand circus can take the wanderlust out of a theatre technician seems ironic, but the employee wellness considerations, among other factors, had that impact.

Utah Shakespeare Festival

For a long time, the Utah Shakespeare Festival (USF) functioned on a weekly stipend basis. During this period, the labor costs were essentially fixed. The work hours were typically 60 hours per week then upwards toward 80 or 100 hours during tech weeks.

This changed in 2013 when the company shifted from a paid stipend model to an hourly wage model. Work weeks were budgeted at 40 to 45 hours per week, but the workload did not significantly change. This meant that anywhere from 20 to 60 hours of overtime was paid, and the company started running a deficit.

Nils Emerson began working as a stage crew supervisor at USF in 2015. The anticipated workload at the time depended on which phase of production the company was in. There were a few weeks of 40–50 hours for preparation, but once into tech, the schedule intensified to a contiguous three 100-hour weeks in a row. Area heads might stay for as many as 140 hours during tech weeks. This was due to dozens of hours sitting tech as well as many hours completing notes and working on other shows when not in tech.

The day-to-day reality of a 100-hour week during tech was arduous. It meant routinely staying late to change scenery (3:00–4:00 a.m.) and then running home to take a nap. Nils would then need to prep for rehearsals starting at 10 a.m. The stage managers would come in at 11:00 a.m., and rehearsals began at noon. There would be brief pockets of time before a run in the evening. Nils would attend the run, stay late, and repeat the cycle.

Working from 10:00 a.m. to 3:00 or 4:00 a.m. the following day was difficult to say the least. Nils would try to "work 'til everything was done," but it was never "done." Nils had issues sorting the daily schedule for the rest of the crew due to his exhaustion. He was not documenting well, as he felt less nimble-minded. Furthermore, he could not optimize his time off; he found himself eating out more often (because who has time to cook?) and drinking beer as a form of recovery. This more costly lifestyle all but negated the benefits of earning extra income through overtime.

Nils was not alone. The workplace exhaustion was also felt by the crew. Despite being paid hourly, there reached a point where many felt the money was just not worth it. When complaints were voiced, a common response at USF was: "Well we're all working a lot, so step in." Other departments felt this way as well. The carpentry morale had also dropped to the point that the crew threatened to walk off the job. This led to a deeply negative view of the season, which affected retention. Very few of the crew returned for the following season, and almost no carpenters returned.[3]

Becky Merold had worked with the USF since 2003. She spent most of her years there working as a stage manager until she took the position of production manager, which she held from 2015 to 2019.

Becky jumped into the production manager position with both feet during the 2015 season. As a stage manager, Becky had not worked anywhere near the hours the crew were working, but as a production manager, she was pulling 100-hour weeks. This started to impact her quality of work.

Becky started having difficulty focusing. She found it challenging to run meetings and remember facts and details, despite normally having a good memory. Her motivation dropped, despite a deep desire to do well in her new position. Changes were jarring and hard to deal with. Any problem that arose put her on the brink of a personal meltdown. Becky recalled crying in the bathroom over these stressors during the first two years in her position.

In 2016, Southern Utah University built a new $40 million-dollar performance center that USF was slated to use for its season. Unfortunately, the center was not yet done when the season started. Nils, newly hired as an assistant technical director, and the technical director worked concurrently on building the productions and finishing the theatre. Everyone pitched in; even the Box Office staff were painting. USF usually went dark on Sunday, but during that process there was a call every Sunday.

Combined with a customarily busy summer schedule, 2016 turned out to be another difficult season. A deck carpenter quit early in the season because of the hours. From the start of her position to the end of 2016, Becky had gained 40 pounds, stopped exercising, and started stress eating and drinking.

However, Becky had learned from the difficult 2015 season, and so during 2016 she and the other department heads tracked their time. By the end of the 2016 season, they had gathered lots of data about their actual working hours.

After the last production of 2016 closed, Becky came to the conclusion that the production model was not sustainable, and so she approached upper management. She brought her actual working hours data and explained the labor situation and its impact. At first, management was incredulous: "But that means you only slept three to four hours per night."

Becky replied: "Yes, we did."

Despite the initial hesitation, upper management accepted that change was necessary. Becky started by analyzing what every show had spent versus what was budgeted. She looked over the previous ten years. She then compared each season and made a discovery.

For USF, Becky found the correlation between labor and material costs, for every department except Wigs, was 3:1.[4] Becky also successfully established that a show was not in budget until both material monies and labor monies were accounted for.

This made it easier not only to project the budgets for a production but also to negotiate. A conversation went from "I really like that, let's drum up another $2000" to then include "but I need another carpenter to do that." It became common knowledge that, if the production wanted to add money to budgets, there would be a labor impact. Becky put it succinctly: "Materials won't just build themselves."

Of course, there were exceptions. Purchasing a prefabricated drop, for example, would not involve much labor to install it. At USF, such a purchase would therefore become a design parameter.

To illustrate this, imagine that *Joseph and the Amazing Technicolor Dreamcoat* has a $5,000 materials need. By applying the USF 3:1 labor ratio, we calculate a $15,000 labor need. The $20,000 overall exceeds the $17,000 show's budget. The team decides to cut a carpenter ($3,000 for the sake of this example) to reduce labor costs, but they leave the materials budget as it is. To do this while still honoring the 3:1 labor-to-materials ratio requires some calculation:

- $15,000 in labor minus $3,000 is $12,000.
- $12,000 divided by three (the USF ratio) is $4,000.
- $5,000 (the materials allocation) minus $4,000 (the appropriate material allocation given the labor allocation) is $1,000.

This means that $1,000 worth of the design must be allocated to a prefabricated, low-labor element, such as curtains or a vinyl drop. This parameter was usually conveyed by the production manager, though it could just as easily have come from artistic leadership.

In the fall of 2017, Nils was hired on full time as the scenery director. He felt fortunate in that his predecessors had begun transforming the labor estimate and construction system. He credited Emily Erdman, the previous scenery director, and Brian Swanson, a seasoned technical director and educator, for integrating the notion of labor costs into production at the carpentry crew level. Nils refined the element-based estimates, accounting for transportation, raw material, and anything else that affected a piece of scenery.

The shop allocated a section in the construction drawings for tracking work hours (down to the nearest half hour), and the crew filled it in as they worked on an element. The diligent tracking of hours yielded two benefits. First, the department had a stronger voice in explaining the value of labor to the creative team; saying "I don't know if we have time to do that" is very different when there is data to support the claim. Second, over the course of several years, the shop got a clearer and clearer picture of how long different processes took. This helped streamline the estimation process.

Beyond labor tracking, Becky also set a hard limit of 80 work hours during tech weeks. Initially, the department heads pushed back. They knew that they were not going to get more labor, and so they were concerned about finishing the shows with fewer hours to jump in and help.

Becky identified that a big draw on time was the need to sit in the theatre during the tech process. To rectify this, she established a new rule: only one person must sit in tech, and everyone else is on call. This made sense, as most notes during tech are not immediately dealt with but rather, left to a notes call later on.

Becky and/or her assistant ended up sitting tech and taking notes for the team. This freed up the department heads to do notes and continue build on other shows, mitigating the loss of work hours under the new 80-hour cap. The only exception would be if there was a big department-specific element going into play. For example, if Becky knew it was going to be an automation-heavy day, she would bring in the technical director to observe the integration.

This was more sustainable for Becky as well. Despite the long hours of tech, she did not need to come in during the morning and would use an afternoon break to take a nap.

Staffing for 2017 was difficult, as word had gotten around that the USF was a difficult place to work. That said, after the season, they found that the new policy improved conditions. For comparison, between 2015 and 2017, scene shop retention was between 30 and 40 percent. Between 2017 and 2019, the shop hit 80 percent crew retention. This meant more skilled staff and a shop that worked more efficiently.

Having worked within a more consistent and mindful schedule, Nils reported that he never wanted to work a "brutal" schedule again. "Put your hand in a fire, and you learn not to do that again." Nils was committed to doing all the preplanning required to avoid "martyring myself on the altar of theater."

After three years, Becky was still feeling the physical impact of her overwork in 2015 and 2016. Despite exercising again, she was not at her ideal weight. She was also dealing with back issues from the overwork. When asked if she would work 100-hour weeks again, perhaps at a more high-paying position, Becky said she didn't think she could.

Works Cited

Kelly, David and Sam Quinones. "Engineer Led Solitary Life Marked by Tragedy." *Los Angeles Times*, 17 September 2008.

Merold, Becky. Interview. Brian Smallwood. 2019.

Smallwood, Brian. *Increasing Productivity Through Employee Wellness*. Thesis, 2013.

Notes

1 (Kelly and Quinones)
2 There is a set limit for the reimbursement, and this benefit is available once per quarter. Other terms and conditions for the arrangement are unavailable to the author at the time of this writing.
3 It should be noted that the Props and Costumes departments had fewer retention issues. It should also be noted that those departments set a 40-hour limit for their staff. If more hours were required, the department heads would step in to pick up the slack.
4 Due to the fact that the raw material in the Wigs department is much cheaper, the ratio in the Wigs department between labor and material cost was 8:1.

Conclusion

By now, my hope is that your view of the production process is a little sharper.

The facts in the "Working" section established that the issue of burnout and work–life balance is affecting our industry. It should also serve as a call for more specific and pointed industry research to better assess the root causes in the live entertainment field.

The consequences of ignoring burnout could be the loss of talent to industries with better work–life practices. As the South Eastern Theatre Conference panel entitled "Where have all the TDs gone?" suggests, the trend is likely already underway.

The "Motivation" section shared a variety of techniques used to make work worth doing. There is a lot of room for experimentation and exploration in terms of sustaining passionate employees. Perhaps these factors are a springboard to a new production approach.

There should be less mystery regarding the "Human Body." Hopefully, the section will inspire personal awareness and make room for moments of decision making when the going gets tough.

"Managing the Work" provided perspective and tools to tackle the ephemeral production process and understand the components at play.

The shared stories in the "Case Studies" section established that innovation is possible, and that increasing productivity and combatting burnout in the workplace is both feasible and a shared interest.

I now charge you, the reader, to advance the conversation. If you vehemently disagree with any of these approaches, discuss why they will not work in your organization. If you found a deep insight into a snag your organization routinely faces, unpack it further. This book is effectively a snapshot of research that many industries are developing. I encourage you to delve more deeply into the issues that face you and your company, and try to fix them. Then, share your results with others.

At the time of this writing, professionals are discussing the value of the 10-out-of-12 rehearsal. Up-and-coming professionals are turning down overtime in favor of work–life balance. The industry is primed for a new sustainable model that honors the contribution of its work force and so is strengthened by it. Perhaps your inquiry and discussion can be the catalyst.

Index

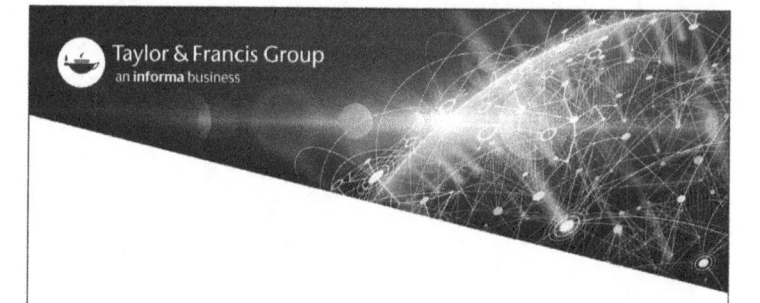
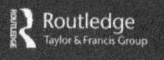
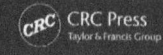